FERMENTED NATURAL COSMETICS

The Power of Microorganisms
**Secret Formulas for
Youthful Skin**

Ava Fiori

Imprint: Independently published
ISBN: 9798325065804

BIOGRAPHY

I am Ava Fiori, an expert with 20 years of experience in the world of natural cosmetics with a special focus on the power of Asian beauty rituals and microorganisms. My professional journey began with a Master's degree in Bioprocess Technology, followed by an in-depth career in product development, marketing, and sales within major corporations in the beauty industry. There, I saw how aggressive chemical ingredients not only provide short-term solutions but also impair skin health in the long term. The promises made by the industry to consumers are often misleading, as chemical creams and care products make the skin dependent and weaken its natural protection.

These insights led me to rethink. Thirteen years ago, I moved to New Zealand, where I came into close contact with a large Asian community and gained deep insights into the traditional care rituals of Korea and Japan. This experience shaped my belief that true beauty and skin health can be achieved through natural, balanced care.

In my ongoing research in the biotechnology industry, I worked closely with microorganisms, especially bacteria, and discovered their incredible potentials for health and skincare. These insights motivated me to share my knowledge and convictions in my book, "Fermented Natural Cosmetics - The Power of Microorganisms: Secret Recipes for Facial Care."
My goal is to enlighten and bridge the gap between traditional wisdom and modern science, to promote natural, effective skincare solutions that are in harmony with our body and nature.

In love with natural beauty

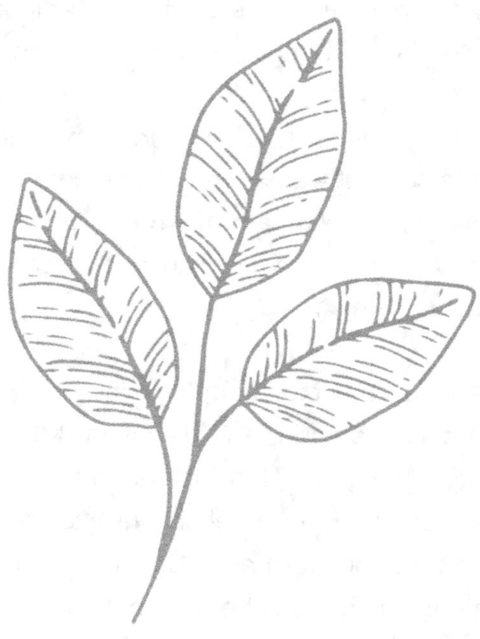

TABLE OF CONTENTS

1. INTRODUCTION

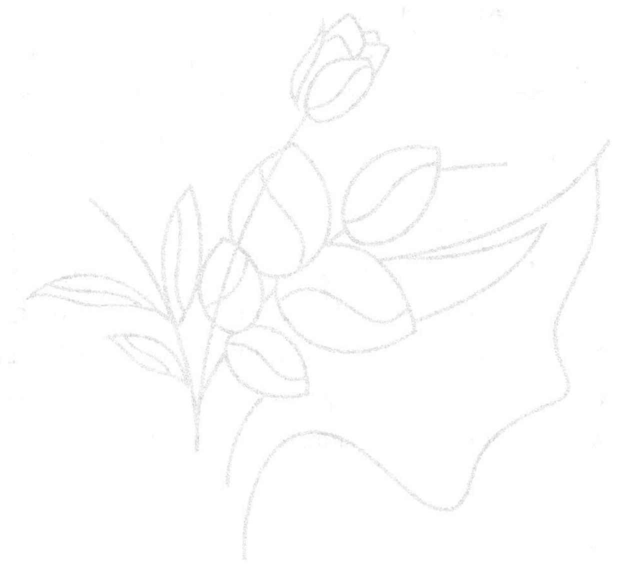

THE MAGIC OF FERMENTED BEAUTY

Have you ever wondered why the skin of Asian women often looks so flawless and youthful, even as the years go by? One well-kept secret of this timeless beauty lies in the traditional use of fermented ingredients in their skincare, a practice that has been common in Asia for centuries.

Fermentation is a biological process where microorganisms like bacteria, yeast and fungi convert organic substances in the absence of oxygen. This wonder of nature has been utilized in the realm of food for decades. However, probiotic and postbiotic ingredients also hold special significance in the realm of outer beauty. For centuries, Asian cultures have been harnessing these valuable components not only for internal health but also for skincare. Although the fermented beauty rituals passed down through generations of Asian women have slowly made their way to the West in recent years, they largely remain a hidden treasure.

Fermented cosmetics are not just a trend but an art form deeply rooted in Asian culture. They serve as a bridge between nature and us, harnessing the power of microorganisms to extract the best from raw materials. In this book, the secrets of fermented cosmetics are unraveled. You'll discover time-tested methods and recipes cherished for generations in Asia. Dive into this world and experience how not only your skin but also your overall well-being can improve.

2. BASICS OF FERMENTATION

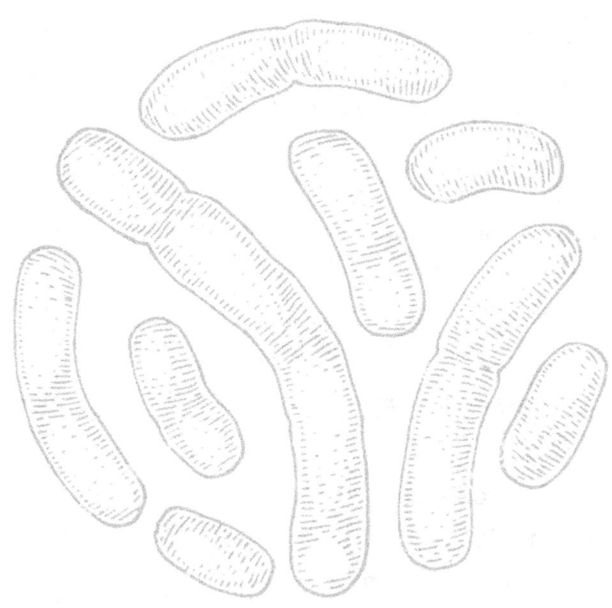

MICROORGANISMS AND THEIR ROLE

At the core of fermentation are microorganisms. These invisible helpers - bacteria, yeasts and sometimes fungi - are responsible for the conversion of organic substances into a variety of end products. In cosmetics, these microorganisms are utilized to transform ingredients that nourish and protect the skin.

Some common microorganisms in fermented cosmetics include:

- **LLactobacillus:** A bacterium commonly found in fermented foods like yogurt. It produces lactic acid, which can balance the skin's pH and act as a gentle exfoliant.

- **Saccharomyces:** A type of yeast used in many skincare products to nourish and hydrate the skin.

- **Bifidobacterium:** Another beneficial bacterium with antioxidant properties that can strengthen the skin barrier.

THE SCIENCE BEHIND FERMENTATION

Fermentation is an anaerobic process, meaning it occurs in the absence of oxygen. During fermentation, microorganisms break down organic substances to gain energy. This process often produces byproducts such as alcohols, gases, or acids.

In cosmetics, this process is utilized to:

- To break down ingredients: Fermentation can break down complex molecules into smaller, more easily absorbable parts. This can increase the bioavailability and effectiveness of an ingredient.

- Creating new compounds: During fermentation, new beneficial compounds can be formed that were not present in the original ingredient. These can have antioxidative, anti-inflammatory, or moisturizing properties.

- Preservation: The acids produced during fermentation can inhibit the growth of harmful microorganisms, thus extending the product's shelf life.

With this understanding of the basics of fermentation, we can now delve deeper into the specific benefits and applications of fermented ingredients in cosmetics.

In the next chapter, we will take a closer look at the various fermented ingredients and their benefits for the skin.

3. BENEFITS OF NATURE

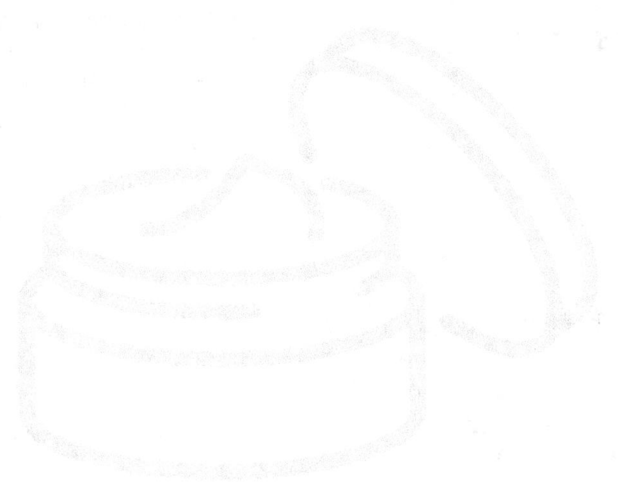

BENEFITS OF FERMENTED INGREDIENTS IN COSMETICS

Fermentation alters the structure and potency of cosmetic ingredients, making them more efficiently absorbed by the skin. This leads to enhanced nutrient delivery and improved results.

Some of the prominent benefits of fermented cosmetics include:

Increased potency

Fermentation can convert many ingredients into their bioactive forms and potentiate some nutrients, enhancing their benefits. For example, ginseng can be transformed into a more potent form through fermentation, rich in active compounds. This results in easier absorption by the skin and more effective action, thus enhancing the overall efficacy of the product.

The acids and other compounds formed during fermentation can inhibit the growth of harmful microorganisms, thus increasing the shelf life of products and reducing the need for synthetic preservatives.

Natural preservation

Promotion of skin health

Some fermented ingredients can positively influence the skin microbiome, contributing to a more robust and healthier skin.

The acids and other compounds formed during fermentation can inhibit the growth of harmful microorganisms, thus increasing the shelf life of products and reducing the need for synthetic preservatives.

Improved absorption and increased bioavailability

Promotion for skin health

Some fermented ingredients can positively influence the skin microbiome, contributing to a more robust and healthier skin.

The fermentation process can create new compounds that were not present in the original plant. These can have antioxidative, anti-inflammatory, or other beneficial properties.

New compounds

In summary, fermented cosmetics combine the benefits of nature with scientific innovations to create powerful and nutrient-rich skincare products.

In the next chapter, we will delve deeper into the fundamentals of fermentation and illuminate the scientific mechanisms behind this impressive process.

4. PLANT EXTRACTS

UNIQUE FERMENTED INGREDIENTS

Before delving into the fascinating world of recipes for fermented cosmetic products, it is crucial to understand the underlying ingredients. Each component has its own story, effects and applications. In the following sections, we will therefore delve deeply into each ingredient, highlighting its benefits and characteristics and provide you with hints and recipes to make the most of these natural wonders. This way, you'll be well-prepared when it comes to creating your own fermented cosmetic products.

FERMENTED PLANT EXTRACTS

Fermented plant extracts are plant materials that have been processed through a fermentation process with the help of microorganisms such as bacteria or yeasts. This process can alter the properties of the original plant material and enhance its benefits for skincare or nutrition.

How are plant extracts fermented?

- **Selection of plant material:** First, a plant material is chosen to be fermented. This could be ginseng, green tea, soybeans, or any other plant with healing or nourishing properties.

- **Addition of microorganisms:** Specific microorganisms, often in the form of starter cultures, are added to the plant material. These microorganisms are responsible for the fermentation process.

- **Fermentation process:** The plant material is then fermented for a specific period at controlled temperatures. During this process, the microorganisms break down certain components of the material and produce new compounds.

- **Extraction:** After fermentation, a solvent (such as water, alcohol, or oil) is used to extract the valuable compounds from the fermented plant material. The resulting product is the fermented plant extract.

Examples of fermented plant extracts

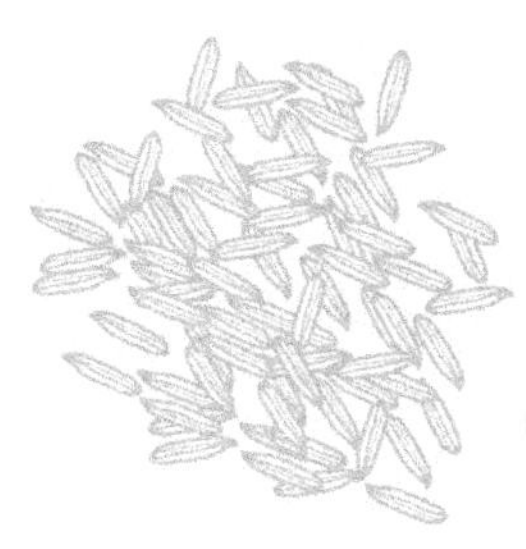

Fermented rice extract

Fermentation enhances the ability of rice extract to balance skin tone and deeply hydrate the skin. Through this process, the ingredients are optimized to promote skin radiance and impart a more even appearance.

Fermented lavender extract

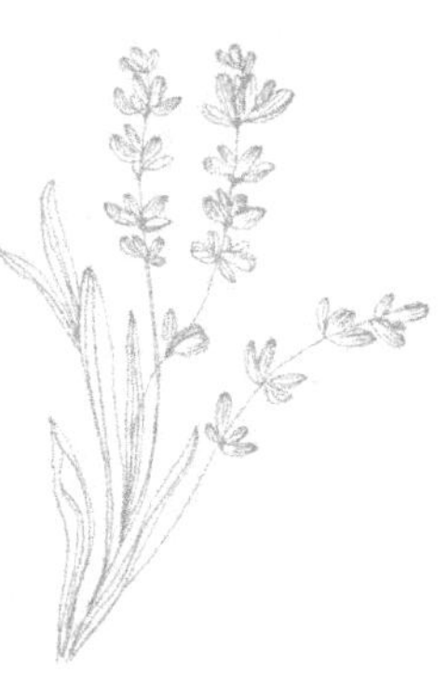

Fermentation enhances the soothing properties of lavender, optimizing its benefits for skincare. This process intensifies lavender's positive effects on the skin by contributing to calming and promoting overall skin well-being.

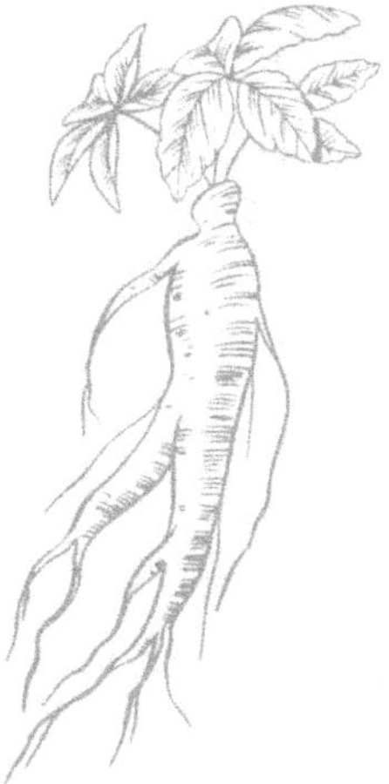

Fermented ginseng extract

Through fermentation, the revitalizing properties of ginseng are enhanced, particularly its antioxidative and anti-aging benefits. This process optimizes the efficacy of ginseng to effectively protect the skin from premature aging and impart a more youthful appearance.

Fermented chamomile extract

Fermentation can enhance the anti-inflammatory and soothing properties of chamomile.

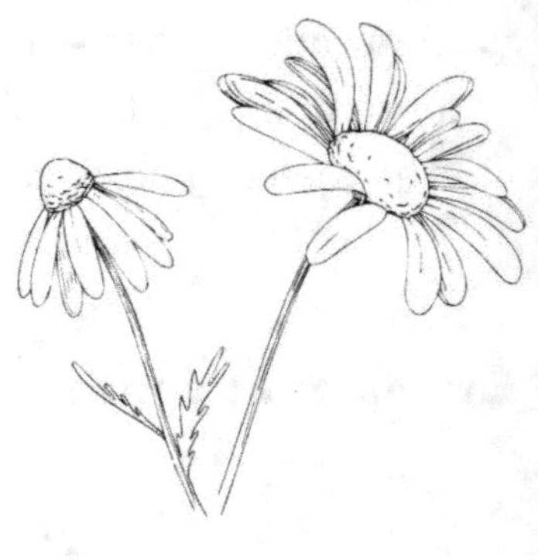

Fermented soybean extract

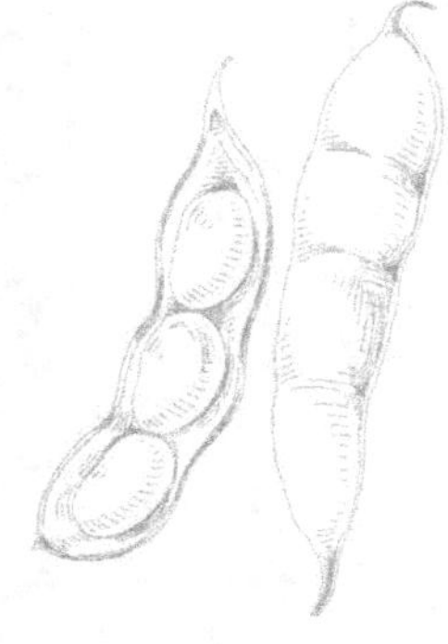

Through fermentation, the properties of soybean extract are enhanced to significantly promote skin elasticity and provide intense hydration. This process helps refine skin texture and increase its suppleness.

Fermented green tea extract

This extract, through fermentation, may contain an increased amount of polyphenols and antioxidants. These substances help the skin protect itself against free radicals - unstable molecules that are created by environmental factors such as sunlight and pollution and can damage skin cells.

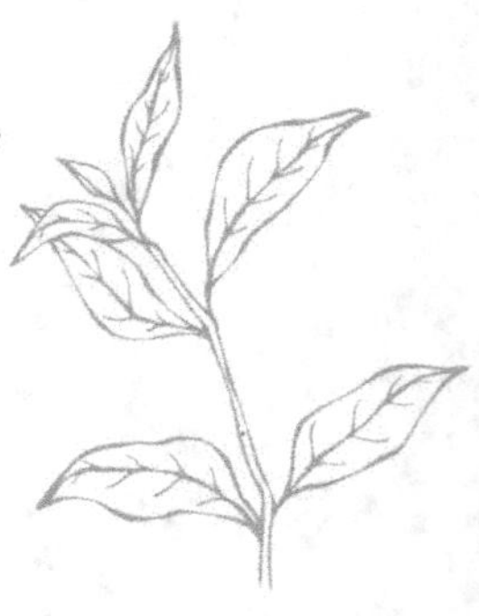

Fermented rose extract

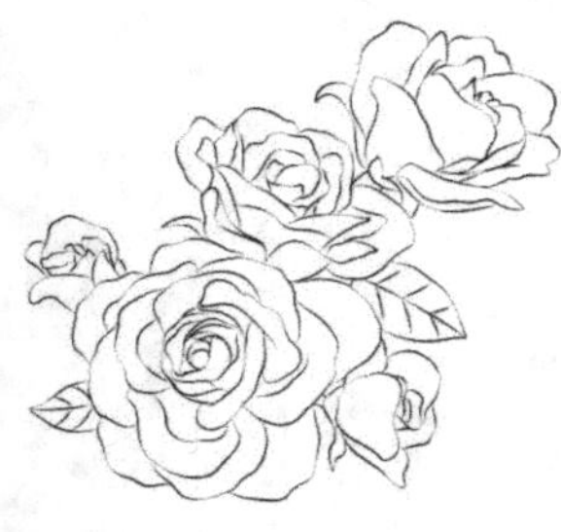

Fermentation enhances the cell-regenerating and antioxidant properties of rose extract. This enhancement supports skin renewal and effectively protects against environmental damage, resulting in a more youthful complexion.

Fermented bamboo extract

Through the fermentation process, the moisturizing and soothing properties of bamboo extract are enhanced. This optimizes its ability to nourish the skin and alleviate redness and irritation.

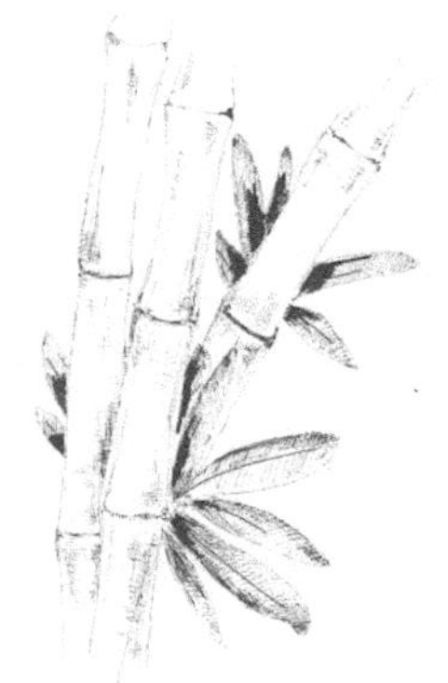

Fermented seaweed extract

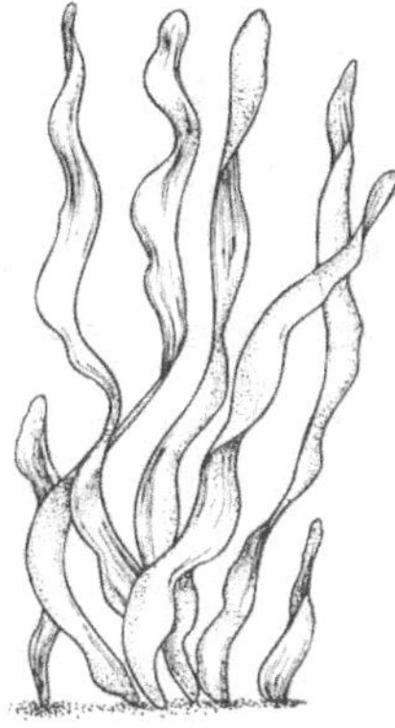

Fermentation enhances the firming and tightening properties of seaweed extract, enriched with a wealth of minerals and vitamins. This process maximizes the positive effects on skin elasticity and supports a healthy skin barrier.

Fermented pomegranate extract

Fermentation optimizes the soothing, hydrating, and tone-balancing properties of pomegranate extract. This enhancement helps to calm the skin, intensely moisturize and promote a more even skin tone.

Ready-to-buy fermented extracts

Fermented extracts can be made at home or purchased ready-made. For those who prefer not to make the extracts themselves due to time constraints, online shops on specialized natural skincare websites, as well as platforms like iHerb and other online retailers, offer a wide range of options. Health food stores with skincare sections and pharmacies specializing in natural products also carry these extracts. Some manufacturers also offer their products directly on their own websites.

If you're willing to venture into creating fermented extracts and ingredients yourself, detailed recipes for your homemade cosmetics await you in the next chapter. However, before exploring the recipes, a brief insight into the role of sugar in the fermentation process is essential to better understand its targeted use.

THE ROLE OF SUGAR IN FERMENTATION:

You might be wondering why the use of sugar is recommended in these recipes, especially considering that sugar is often viewed critically for both internal consumption and external application. However, it's crucial to recognize the central role sugar plays in numerous fermentation processes.

Sugar serves as a key energy source for the bacteria and yeasts essential for initiating and maintaining fermentation. It functions as:

- **Energy source for microorganisms:** During fermentation, microorganisms, mainly yeasts and bacteria, consume sugar as an energy source. This process is known as glycolysis.

- **Production of byproducts:** As these microorganisms metabolize sugar, they produce byproducts such as alcohol, gases (e.g., carbon dioxide), and acids (e.g., lactic acid). These byproducts, especially the acids, are often the desired end products of fermentation. They not only impart the characteristic taste and aroma of fermented products but also possess preserving properties. Additionally, they lower the product's pH, which can be beneficial for the skin, effectively inhibiting the growth of unwanted bacteria and molds. Moreover, some of these end products such as hyaluronic acid, lactic acid, vitamins, peptides, proteins, kojic acid and antioxidants are of particular interest in cosmetics. They are valued for their moisturizing, exfoliating, antioxidant, and skin-brightening properties.

No need to worry about the sugar in the end product: For those concerned about the sugar content in their cosmetics, it's important to understand that the sugar originally added for fermentation is barely present in the final product. During the fermentation process, the majority of the sugar is consumed by the microorganisms and converted into the aforementioned byproducts such as alcohol, gases (e.g., carbon dioxide) and acids (e.g., lactic acid). This means that in the final product, there is very little, if any, original sugar left.

5.DIY RECIPES FERMENTED PLANT EXTRACTS

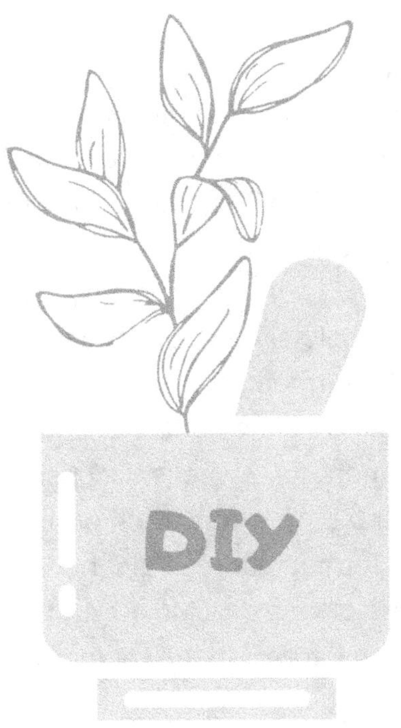

FERMENTED GINSENG EXTRACT

An elixir for radiant skin, Ginseng, often referred to as the "root of life," has been revered in many Asian cultures for centuries for its healing and rejuvenating properties. Fermented Ginseng Extract amplifies these benefits and can be used as a potent serum for the skin or as an additive to other skincare products.

Ingredients:
- 60 g fresh Ginseng
- 100 g distilled water
- 6 g white sugar
- A clean glass container with lid

Instructions for preparation:
1. Preparation of Ginseng: Wash the ginseng thoroughly under running water to remove any dirt or residue. Then, slice it into thin, uniform slices.
2. Place the ginseng slices into the glass container.
3. Add the sugar, using about 10% of the total weight of the ginseng as a guideline.
4. Cover the ginseng completely with distilled water to ensure it is fully submerged during the fermentation process.
5. Fermentation process: Seal the container tightly and place it in a warm, dark place. Let it sit there for 2 weeks. Occasionally check the container to ensure that no unwanted mold formation or other anomalies occur.
6. After completing the fermentation, strain the liquid ginseng extract through a fine sieve. Store the clear extract in a clean container. For optimal freshness and potency, store it in the refrigerator and use it within 2-3 weeks.

Note: As with all fermented products, the smell of the ginseng extract may be strong and earthy. This is a sign that the fermentation was successful. However, if you detect any unpleasant or rotten smell, discard the extract and start over.

FERMENTED GREEN TEA EXTRACT

Green tea is globally recognized for its antioxidant and anti-inflammatory properties. Through fermentation, these benefits are further enhanced, creating a powerful elixir that protects your skin from harmful radicals and gives it a youthful glow.

Ingredients:
- 40 g high-quality green tea
- 100 g distilled water
- 4 g white sugar
- A clean glass container with a lid

Instructions for preparation:
1. Preparation of the tea: Place the loose green tea in the glass container. The quality of the tea is crucial as it constitutes the main ingredient of the extract.
2. Add the sugar, using approximately 10% of the total weight of the tea as a guideline.
3. Cover the tea completely with distilled water to ensure it is fully submerged during the fermentation process.
4. Fermentation process: Seal the container tightly and place it in a warm, dark place. Let it sit there for 1-2 weeks. Occasionally check the container to ensure no unwanted mold formation or other anomalies occur.
5. After the fermentation is complete, strain the liquid green tea extract through a fine sieve. Store the clear extract in a clean container. For optimal freshness and potency, store it in the refrigerator and use it within 2-3 weeks.

Note: A slightly sour smell indicates that the fermentation was successful. However, if you detect an unpleasant or foul odor, it suggests that something went wrong. In this case, discard the extract and start the process again.

FERMENTED LAVENDER EXTRACT

Lavender, with its distinctive scent and soothing properties, holds a firm place in aromatherapy and skincare. Fermented lavender extract combines the calming benefits of lavender with the power of fermentation to provide deeper skin nourishment and relaxation.

Ingredients:
- 20 g fresh lavender flowers
- 100 ml distilled water
- 2 g white sugar
- A glass container with a lid

Instructions for preparation:
1. The lavender flowers carefully plucked from the stems and placed into the glass container.
2. Add sugar (about 10% of the weight of the lavender).
3. Cover with distilled water.
4. Fermentation process: Seal the container and let it sit in a warm, dark place for 1-2 weeks.
5. After fermentation is complete, strain the liquid lavender extract through a fine sieve. Store the clear extract in a clean container. For optimal freshness and potency, store in the refrigerator and use within 2-3 weeks.

Note: The fermented lavender extract may develop an intensified, soothing lavender scent, which is a clear sign of successful fermentation. However, if an unusually strong or unpleasant odor occurs, it is advisable to discard the extract and start the fermentation process again.

FERMENTED KOMBU EXTRACT (SEAWEED)

Kombu, an essential ingredient in Asian cuisine, is not only nutritious for the body but also beneficial for the skin. As a fermented extract, Kombu provides a wealth of minerals and vitamins that help the skin retain moisture and improve its elasticity.

Ingredients:
- 10 g dried Kombu (kelp)
- 100 ml distilled water
- 1 g white sugar
- A glass container with a lid

Instructions for preparation:
1. Soak the Kombu in cold water for about 10-15 minutes until it softens.
2. Remove the soaked Kombu from the water and cut it into thin strips.
3. Place the Kombu strips in a clean glass container. Add sugar (about 10% of the weight of the Kombu).
4. Cover with distilled water.
5. Fermentation process: Seal the container and let it sit in a warm, dark place for 1-2 weeks.
6. After fermentation is complete, strain the liquid Kombu extract through a fine sieve. Store the clear extract in a clean container. For optimal freshness and potency, store in the refrigerator and use within 2-3 weeks.

Note: A slightly sour smell indicates successful fermentation. However, if you detect an unpleasant or rotten smell, it suggests something went wrong. In this case, discard the extract and start the process again.

FERMENTED KOJI RICE EXTRACT

Koji rice is rice fermented with a special fungus (Aspergillus oryzae) and serves as the foundation for many Japanese fermented products like Sake, Miso, and Soy Sauce. It contains enzymes that can exfoliate and brighten the skin. Additionally, it offers moisturizing and anti-aging benefits.

Ingredients:
- 100 g cooked white rice
- 2 g koji spores (available in specialty stores or online)
- 100 ml water

Instructions for preparation:
1. Allow cooked white rice to cool.
2. Sprinkle Koji spores over the rice and mix well.
3. Fermentation process: Spread the rice in a shallow container and ferment at a temperature of about 30°C for 36-48 hours. The rice should develop a sweet note and a pleasant fungal aroma.
4. Mix the fermented rice with water and let it stand for 24 hours again.
5. Filtering and storage: After fermentation is complete, filter the liquid Koji rice extract through a fine sieve. Store the clear extract in a clean container. For optimal freshness and potency, store in the refrigerator and use within 2-3 weeks.

Note: The fermented koji rice extract may develop a characteristic sweet and pleasantly mushroomy scent, which is an indicator of successful fermentation. If you notice an unusually strong or unpleasant odor, it is advisable to discard the extract and start the fermentation process again.

FERMENTED JUJUBE EXTRACT (RED DATE)

Red dates, also known as Jujubes, are highly valued in Traditional Chinese Medicine (TCM) and are often used in tonics. They are renowned for their soothing and nourishing properties. Jujube extract intensely moisturizes, calms the skin and can reduce redness. Additionally, it is rich in vitamins and minerals that revitalize the skin.

Ingredients:
- 100 g fresh red dates (Jujubes)-available online or at Asian grocery stores
- 10 g white sugar (approximately 10% of the weight of the red dates)
- 100 ml distilled water
- A clean glass container with a lid

Instructions for preparation:
1. Wash and pit the fresh red dates.
2. Slice the red dates thinly and place them in a clean glass container.
3. Cover with distilled water and add the sugar.
4. Fermentation process: Seal the container and let it ferment at room temperature for 7-10 days.
5. Filter and store: After fermentation is complete, strain the liquid Jujube extract through a fine sieve.
6. Store the clear extract in a clean container. For optimal freshness and potency, store in the refrigerator and use within 2-3 weeks.

Note: The fermented Jujube (Red Date) extract may develop a sweet, pleasant aroma, which is a sign of successful fermentation. However, if an unusually strong or unpleasant odor is noticed, it is advisable to discard the extract and start the fermentation process anew.

FERMENTED CHAMOMILE EXTRACT

Chamomile extract, derived from the delicate flowers of the chamomile plant, has long been recognized for its soothing and anti-inflammatory properties. Chamomile is often used in skincare to calm and nourish sensitive skin. Fermented chamomile extract enhances these beneficial effects and can serve as a key ingredient in cosmetic recipes for sensitive skin.

Ingredients:
- 20 g dried chamomile flowers
- 200 g distilled water
- 1 g white sugar
- A clean glass container with a lid

Instructions for preparation:
1. Place the dried chamomile flowers in the clean glass container.
2. Slightly warm the distilled water until it is lukewarm, then pour it over the chamomile flowers.
3. Add the sugar and mix everything well. Close the container with a lid.
4. Fermentation process: Let the mixture ferment in a warm place for about 48 hours. During this time, the fermented chamomile extract will develop.
5. After fermentation, strain the liquid through a fine sieve or coffee filter to remove the chamomile flower residue.
6. Transfer the liquid fermented chamomile extract to a clean glass container with a lid. Make sure to store it in a cool place and use it within 2-4 weeks.

Note: The fermented chamomile extract may develop a mild, pleasant scent, indicating successful fermentation. However, if an unusually strong or unpleasant odor develops, it is advisable to discard the extract and start the fermentation process again.

FERMENTED BLACK RICE EXTRACT

Fermented black rice extract is a potent ingredient in Asian skincare, nurturing the skin in various ways. It's rich in antioxidants, including anthocyanins, which shield the skin from free radicals, counteracting premature aging. This antioxidative effect helps diminish wrinkles and fine lines, while its moisturizing properties ensure deep hydration, leaving the skin soft and supple. Moreover, the extract can brighten the complexion, reduce pigmentation spots, soothe redness and irritation and strengthen the skin barrier, making it more resilient against environmental stressors.

Ingredients:
- 100 g uncooked black rice
- 10 g white sugar (approximately 10% of the rice weight)
- 100 ml distilled water
- A clean glass container with a lid

Instructions for preparation:
1. Wash the black rice thoroughly.
2. Cover the rice with distilled water in a glass container. Add sugar and stir well.
3. Fermentation process: Seal the container tightly and place it in a warm, dark place for 5-7 days. Check the progress occasionally to ensure no mold or other unwanted reactions occur.
4. Filter and store: After fermentation is complete, filter the liquid extract through a fine sieve.
5. Store the clear extract in a clean container. For optimal freshness and effectiveness, store the extract in the refrigerator and use it within 2-3 weeks.

Note: The fermented black rice extract may have an intense but pleasant aroma, which is an indicator of successful fermentation. However, if an unusually strong or unpleasant odor occurs, it is advisable to discard the extract and start the process anew.

FERMENTED SOYBEAN EXTRACT (CHEONGGUKJANG)

Cheonggukjang, known in Korean cuisine as "fast-fermented soybean paste," is characterized by its intense fermentation and distinctive flavor. In skincare, the water resulting from the fermentation process is valued for its nourishing and revitalizing properties. It is rich in isoflavones, which can help reduce signs of aging. Additionally, Cheonggukjang offers antioxidant benefits that protect the skin from harmful free radicals and may help harmonize skin tone and refine skin texture.

Ingredients:
- 200 grams raw soybeans
- 400 grams water
- 1 teaspoon fermentation starter (e.g., Bacillus subtilis)
- A clean container with a lid

Instructions for preparation:
1. Soak raw soybeans in water overnight.
2. Cook the beans until they are soft, then let them cool. Transfer the cooked beans to a clean container and add a fermentation starter (e.g., Bacillus subtilis, available at some Asian grocery stores).
3. Fermentation process: Allow the beans to ferment at room temperature for 3-5 days.
4. They should develop a strong odor typical of Cheonggukjang.
5. Filter and store: After fermentation is complete, filter the liquid extract through a sieve. Store the clear extract in a clean container.
6. For optimal freshness and effectiveness, store the extract in the refrigerator and use it within 2-3 weeks.

Important: Fermentation Starter - See next page

Fermentation starter / Fermentation culture

- The use of a fermentation starter depends on the specific type of fermentation and the desired results. In some recipes, such as the one for Fermented Bean Sprout Water Extract (Cheonggukjang), a fermentation starter like Bacillus subtilis is used to expedite the fermentation process and ensure that the desired microorganisms are active.

- In other recipes, such as those for fermented extracts from rice, tea, or lavender, fermentation occurs more naturally through the microorganisms already present on the ingredients or developed during the fermentation process. In these cases, no additional fermentation starter is required.

- The decision to use a fermentation starter depends on traditional practices and desired outcomes and not all fermented extracts necessitate a starter. It's important to carefully follow the instructions in each recipe and adhere to the recommended ingredients and steps to achieve the desired results.

Ready-to-buy fermented extracts

The fermentation starter, such as Bacillus subtilis, is typically available in specialized stores for fermented foods or online from providers of fermented food ingredients. It's important to ensure that the fermentation starter used is suitable for consumption or skincare. Follow the manufacturer's instructions for the proper use and storage of the starter.

FERMENTED ROSE EXTRACT

Roses, cherished in cosmetics for centuries for their nourishing and soothing properties, offer a true treasure trove of benefits. Fermented rose extract enhances these beneficial effects, making the skin supple and imparting a radiant appearance.

Ingredients:
- 50 g fresh red or pink rose petals (Rosa damascena or Rosa centifolia)
- 100 ml distilled water
- 5 g white sugar
- A clean glass container with a lid

Instructions for preparation:
1. Rinse the rose petals gently under running water to remove any dirt.
2. Place the cleaned rose petals into the glass container.
3. Sprinkle the sugar over the rose petals, using about 10% of the weight of the rose petals as a guideline.
4. Water addition: Pour the distilled water over the rose petals, ensuring they are fully covered.
5. Fermentation process: Seal the container and let it sit in a warm, dark place for 1 week.
6. Check occasionally to ensure no mold develops.
7. Filtering and storage: Strain the finished rose extract and store it in a clean container. Keep it in the refrigerator and use it within 2-3 weeks.

Note: The fermented rose extract may develop an intensely floral scent, which is considered a sign of successful fermentation. However, if an unusually strong or unpleasant odor is detected, it is advisable to discard the extract and start the fermentation process again.

FERMENTED BAMBOO EXTRACT

Bamboo, known for its moisturizing and healing properties, is a wonder ingredient for the skin. Fermented bamboo extract harnesses these natural benefits to deeply hydrate the skin and improve its elasticity.

Ingredients:
- 60 g fresh bamboo shoots (no canned bamboo! Available at Asian grocery stores or online)
- 100 ml distilled water
- 6 g white sugar
- A clean glass container with a lid

Instructions for preparation:
1. Prepare the bamboo shoots: Peel and slice the bamboo shoots thinly.
2. Place the bamboo shoots in the glass container.
3. Add the sugar. Cover the shoots completely with distilled water.
4. Fermentation process: Let the container sit in a warm, dark place for 1 week.
5. Filter and store: Strain the finished bamboo extract and store it in a clean container.
6. Store in the refrigerator and use within 2-3 weeks.

Note: A characteristic, fresh scent indicates that the fermented bamboo extract has successfully fermented. However, if you detect a strong or unusual odor that does not match the expected fresh and slightly sweet aroma, you should discard the extract and repeat the fermentation process.

FERMENTED POMEGRANATE EXTRACT

Pomegranate, rich in antioxidants, supports skin regeneration and combats signs of aging. Fermented pomegranate extract enhances these effects for vibrant and youthful-looking skin.

Ingredients:
- 100 g fresh pomegranate seeds
- 100 ml distilled water
- 10 g white sugar
- A clean glass container with a lid

Instructions for preparation:
1. Prepare the pomegranate seeds: Remove the seeds from the pomegranate.
2. Place the seeds in the glass container.
3. Add the sugar. Pour the distilled water over the seeds, ensuring they are fully covered.
4. Fermentation process: Seal the container tightly and place it in a warm, dark place. Let it ferment for about 1-2 weeks.
5. Check the container occasionally to ensure no unwanted mold formation or other anomalies occur.
6. Filter and store: After fermentation is complete, filter the liquid pomegranate extract through a fine sieve.
7. Store the clear extract in a clean container. For optimal freshness and potency, store in the refrigerator and use within 2-3 weeks.

Note: Fermented pomegranate extract is characterized by a sweet and tangy aroma, indicating successful fermentation. If an unusually intense or unpleasant odor occurs, it is advisable to discard the extract and restart the fermentation process from the beginning.

6.FERMENTED OILS

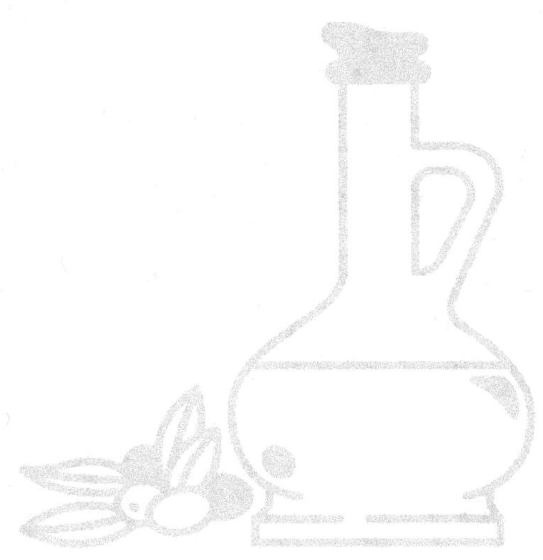

BRIEF INTRODUCTION

Fermented oil refers to oils that have undergone a fermentation process with the assistance of microorganisms such as bacteria or yeasts. This process can alter the properties of the original oil and enhance its benefits for skincare or nutrition.

How is oil fermented?

- **Selection of base oil:** Firstly, a base oil is chosen to undergo fermentation. This can be any vegetable oil such as olive oil, coconut oil, jojoba oil, or argan oil.

- **Addition of microorganisms:** Specific microorganisms, often in the form of starter cultures, are added to the oil. These microorganisms are responsible for the fermentation process.

- **Fermentation process:** The oil is then fermented for a specific duration at controlled temperatures. During this process, the microorganisms break down certain components of the oil and produce new compounds

- **Filtration and storage:** After fermentation, the oil is filtered to remove excess microorganisms and other residues. The resulting fermented oil is then stored in clean containers.

Benefits of fermented oil

New compounds

The fermentation process can generate new compounds that were not present in the original oil source. These may possess antioxidative, anti-inflammatory, or other beneficial properties.

Increased bioavailability

Fermentation can reduce the molecular size of certain components of the oil, making them easier to be absorbed by the skin.

Enhanced nutrients

Some nutrients in the oil can be potentiated through fermentation, enhancing their benefits.

EXAMPLES OF FERMENTED OILS

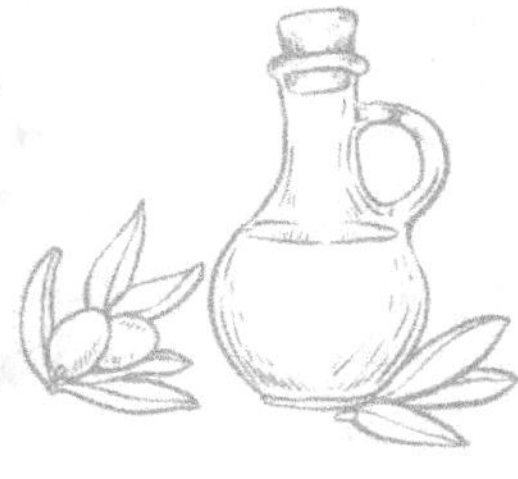

Fermented olive oil

This oil is often valued for its moisturizing properties. Through fermentation, it can be more readily absorbed by the skin, providing deeper hydration.

Fermented coconut oil

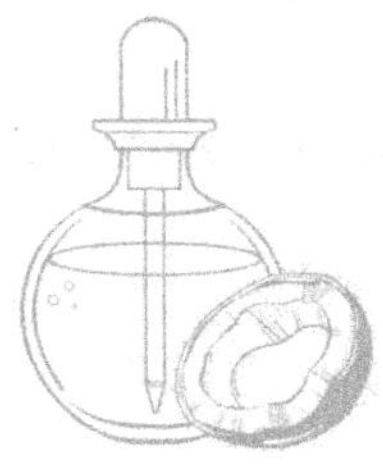

Known for its antimicrobial properties, fermentation can enhance the nutrient availability of coconut oil, making it particularly beneficial for dry or acne-prone skin.

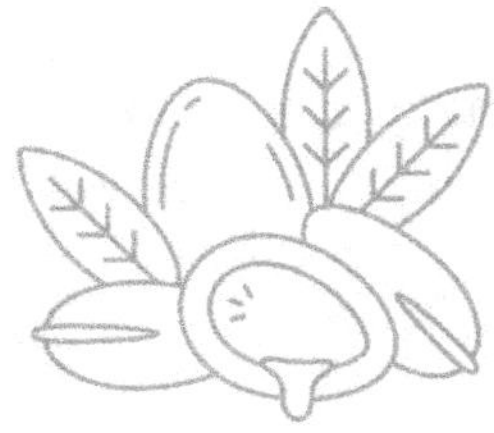

Fermented argan oil

This oil, often referred to as 'liquid gold,' is rich in vitamin E and fatty acids. Fermentation can potentiate its antioxidant properties, making it an excellent choice for anti-aging products.

Fermented jojoba oil

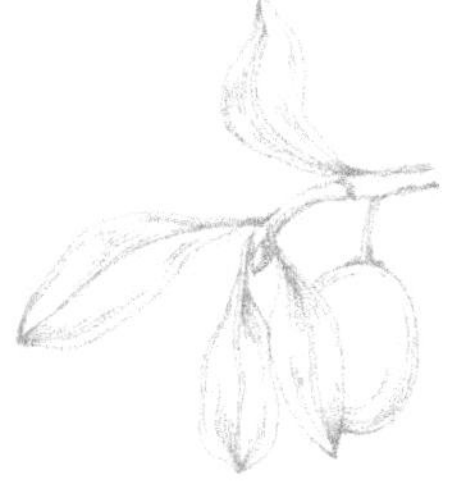

Due to its chemical similarity to human sebum, jojoba oil is particularly compatible with the skin. Fermentation can enhance its anti-inflammatory and healing properties.

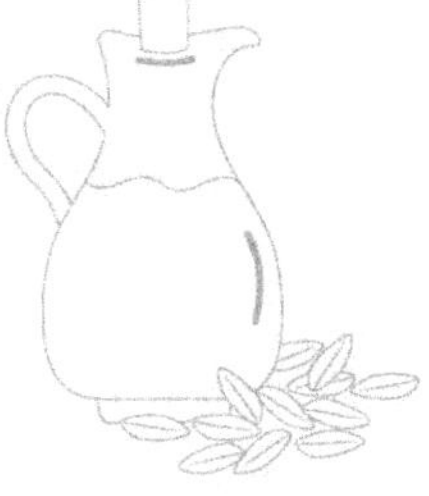

Fermented flaxseed oil

Rich in omega-3 fatty acids, fermented flaxseed oil can help strengthen the skin barrier and reduce inflammation.

Ready-to-buy fermented oils

Fermented oils, like fermented extracts, can be either homemade or purchased ready-made. For those who don't have the time to make the oils themselves, numerous sources offer a wide range of options. Many well-stocked health food stores, specialized online shops like iHerb, stores focusing on natural cosmetics and pharmacies with a focus on natural products carry these extracts. Additionally, some manufacturers of fermented products sell their items directly through their own websites, making it easier to access a variety of options. You can also find local producers of fermented products at fairs and markets, such as organic markets or health expos.

Tips for buying:

- **Read the label:** Make sure the product actually contains fermented ingredients and isn't just using marketing buzzwords.

- **Freshness and shelf life:** Fermented oils can have a limited shelf life, especially if they don't contain preservatives. Check the expiration date and store the oil in the refrigerator after opening if recommended.

- **Origin and quality:** Prefer oils from organic farming and look for certificates or quality seals confirming the origin and production process.

7.DIY RECIPES FERMENTED OILS

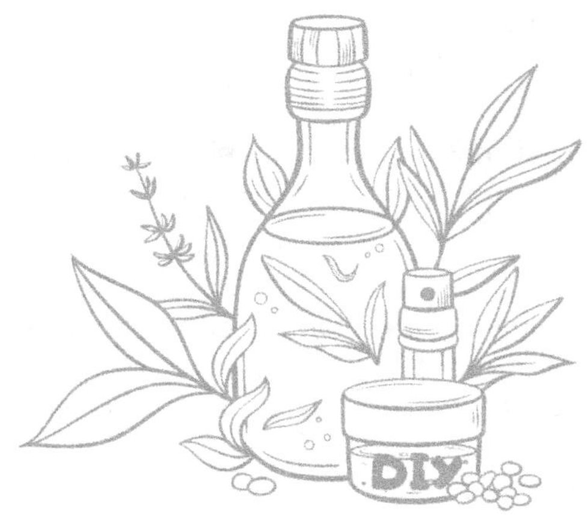

REQUIRED FERMENTATION CULTURES

To produce fermented oils, the addition of a starter culture or starter juice is essential. While fermentation of extracts often relies on the natural microorganisms already present on the plants, oils require external starters due to their purity and lack of water-based components. These starter cultures or juices initiate the fermentation process by providing the necessary microorganisms that do not naturally occur in oils.

Possible starters for fermentation:

- Fermented rice water (see recipe in the book)
- Sauerkraut juice
- Other fermented juices that can serve as starters

Please note that a few drops of the chosen starter juice should be added to the oils. This helps initiate the fermentation process.

Note: When making fermented oils at home, it's important to ensure that all utensils and containers used are clean and sterile. Monitor the fermentation process regularly to ensure that no unwanted microorganisms, such as mold, grow.

FERMENTED OLIVE OIL

Fermented olive oil, enriched with vitamins and antioxidants, provides deep nourishment for the skin. It enhances elasticity, protects against premature skin aging, and leaves the skin feeling smooth. Ideal for daily use to strengthen the skin and give it a radiant appearance.

Ingredients:

- 100 grams of pure olive oil
- A few drops of starter juice
- Clean glass container

Instructions for preparation:

1. Pour the olive oil into a clean glass container.
2. Add a few drops of the starter juice.
3. Seal the container and let it sit at room temperature for 5-7 days.
4. Strain the oil through a fine sieve and store it in a clean container.

FERMENTED COCONUT OIL

Fermented coconut oil nourishes and soothes the skin with its intensely moisturizing properties. Rich in medium-chain fatty acids, it supports the skin's natural barrier function, combats dryness and promotes a healthy complexion. An ideal skincare product for all skin types, providing protection and suppleness.

Ingredients:
- 100 grams of pure coconut oil
- A few drops of starter juice
- Clean glass container

Instructions for preparation:
1. Place the coconut oil into a clean glass container.
2. Add a few drops of the starter juice.
3. Seal the container and let it sit at room temperature for 5-7 days.
4. Strain the oil through a fine sieve and store it in a clean container.

FERMENTED ARGAN OIL

Fermented argan oil, rich in vitamin E and essential fatty acids, provides intensive nourishment and regeneration to the skin. It helps retain moisture, reduce wrinkles and improve skin texture. A valuable oil for revitalizing and protecting the skin, particularly suitable for dry and mature skin types.

Ingredients:

- 100 grams of pure argan oil
- A few drops of starter juice
- Clean glass container

Instructions for preparation:

- Place the argan oil into a clean glass container.
- Add a few drops of the starter juice.
- Seal the container and let it sit at room temperature for 5-7 days.
- Strain the oil through a fine sieve and store it in a clean container.

FERMENTED JOJOBA OIL

Similar to human sebum chemically, jojoba oil is known for its high skin compatibility and versatile skincare properties, including moisturizing without leaving a greasy film, antioxidant protection and regulation of sebum production. It also promotes skin regeneration and strengthens the skin barrier. Fermentation enhances these positive effects further, making jojoba oil particularly valuable for sensitive skin types.

Ingredients:
- 100 grams of pure jojoba oil
- A few drops of starter juice
- Clean glass container

Instructions for preparation:
- Place the jojoba oil into a clean glass container.
- Add a few drops of the starter juice.
- Seal the container and let it sit at room temperature for 5-7 days.
- Strain the oil through a fine sieve and store it in a clean container.

FERMENTED FLAXSEED OIL

Fermented flaxseed oil is a rich source of omega-3 fatty acids, known for their anti-inflammatory properties and ability to strengthen the skin barrier. It helps to alleviate redness and irritation, promotes skin regeneration and provides deep hydration. A true treasure for those looking to naturally nourish and protect their skin.

Ingredients:
- 100 grams of pure flaxseed oil
- A few drops of starter juice
- Clean glass container

Instructions for preparation:
- Place the flaxseed oil into a clean glass container.
- Add a few drops of the starter juice.
- Seal the container and let it sit at room temperature for 5-7 days.
- Strain the oil through a fine sieve and store it in a clean container.

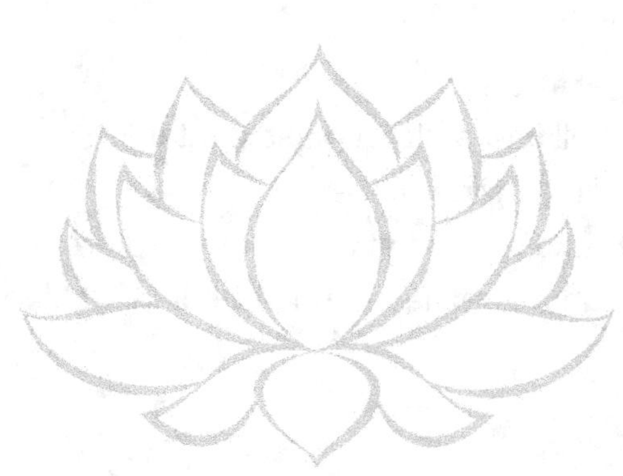

8.FERMENTED DAIRY PRODUCTS

BRIEF INTRODUCTION

Fermented dairy products have been a staple of human nutrition for millennia. By using lactic acid bacteria and other microorganisms, milk sugar (lactose) and other components of milk are converted into lactic acid and other beneficial compounds. This process not only gives the products their characteristic texture and tangy taste but also imparts a range of health benefits.

Benefits for the skin:

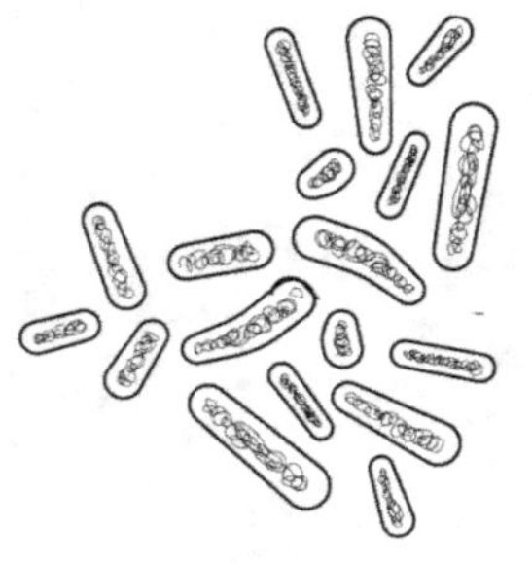

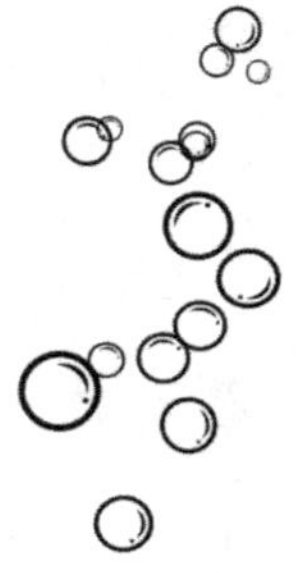

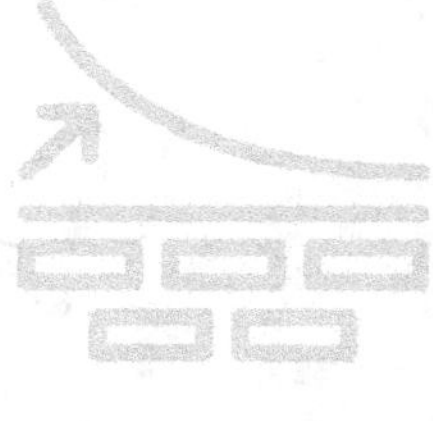

Probiotic Effect

The live cultures found in fermented dairy products can positively influence the skin's microbiome.
A balanced skin microbiome can contribute to a healthier, more resilient skin.

Hydration

The proteins, fats, and natural humectants in fermented dairy products can nourish and hydrate the skin.

Gentle exfoliation

The lactic acid present in fermented dairy products can act as a gentle exfoliant, removing dead skin cells and promoting skin renewal.

EXAMPLES OF FERMENTED DAIRY PRODUCTS

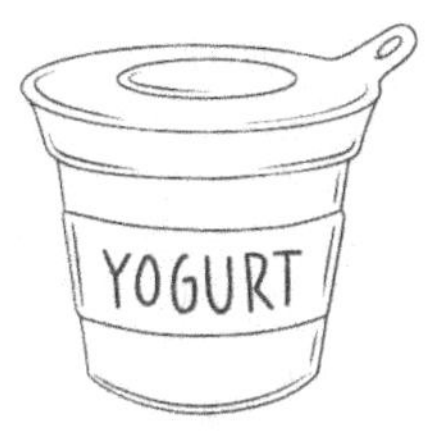

Natural yogurt

A natural probiotic often used in facial masks and cleansers. It can help even out skin tone and soothe the skin.

Kefir

Similar to yogurt but with a greater variety of probiotic cultures. It has anti-inflammatory properties and can help with skin issues such as acne or rosacea.

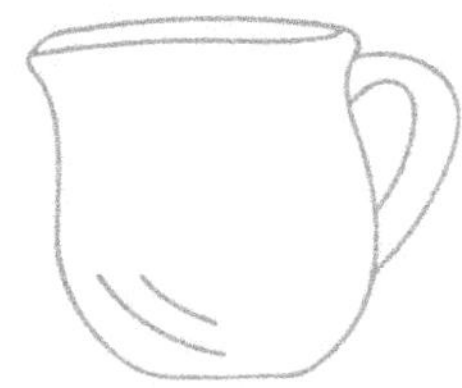

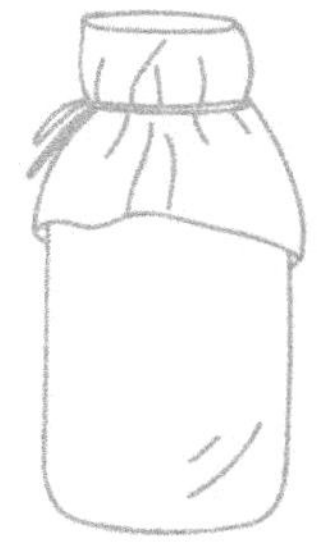

Buttermilk

Contains lactic acid and is often used in peels and masks to renew and smooth the skin.

Ready-to-buy fermented dairy products:

Fermented dairy products are available in most supermarkets and health food stores. For cosmetic purposes, opt for products without additives or sugar. Alternatively, you can make them at home. However, keep in mind that hygiene is of utmost importance when making fermented products at home. Ensure that all utensils and containers are clean and sterilized to minimize the risk of contamination with unwanted microorganisms.

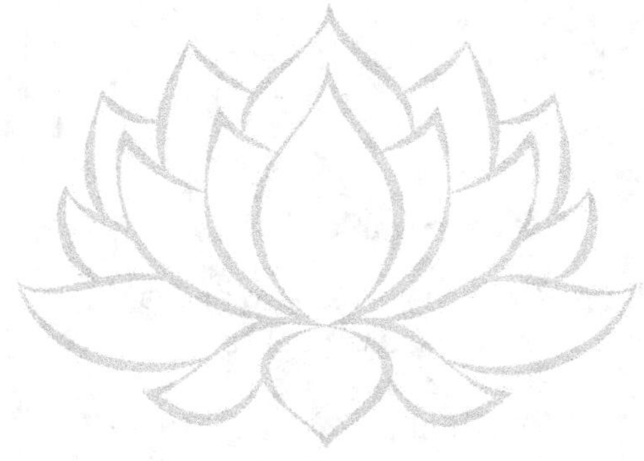

9.DIY RECIPES
FERMENTED DAIRY PRODUCTS

YOGURT

Ingredients:
- 1 liter of whole milk (preferably fresh, not ultra-pasteurized)
- 2 tablespoons of natural yogurt (as a starter culture, make sure "live cultures" are listed on the label) or 2 tablespoons of kefir

Instructions for preparation:

1. Heat the milk in a pot until it is almost boiling (about 85°C). Then remove from heat and let cool to about 43°C.
2. Stir the natural yogurt into the cooled milk.
3. Pour the mixture into clean jars or a yogurt maker.
4. Leave in a warm place for 6-12 hours. An oven with the light on or a yogurt maker are ideal.
5. After fermentation, place the yogurt in the refrigerator. It will firm up after a few hours.

Note:

Storage: Freshly made yogurt should be stored in the refrigerator and will generally keep for about 1 to 2 weeks.

Consistency: If you prefer a firmer yogurt, you can let it ferment longer or strain it through cheesecloth after fermentation to remove the whey.

Smell and Taste: Fresh yogurt should have a pleasantly sour smell and taste. An unpleasant or rotten smell is a sign that the yogurt is no longer good.

KEFIR

Ingredients:
- 1 liter of whole milk
- 1 tablespoon of kefir grains (available in health food stores or online)

Instructions for preparation:
1. Add the kefir grains.
2. Cover with a clean cloth and secure with a rubber band or string.
3. Let stand at room temperature for 12-48 hours, depending on the desired consistency and sourness.
4. Pour the kefir through a sieve to collect the kefir grains.
5. Save the kefir grains for the next batch.

Note:

Storage: Kefir can be stored in the refrigerator after fermentation. Freshly prepared kefir typically lasts about 1 to 2 weeks in the refrigerator. However, it is important to note that kefir will continue to ferment over time, even when chilled, though at a slower rate. This means it will become more sour over time and may also become slightly fizzy or carbonated.

Smell and Taste: Fresh kefir has a sweetly sour taste. If you keep kefir longer, you should regularly check whether it still smells and tastes good. An unpleasant or rotten smell is a sign that the kefir is no longer good and should be discarded.

BUTTERMILK

Ingredients:
- 1 liter of whole milk
- 60 ml cultured buttermilk (available in natural food stores)

Instructions for preparation:
1. Pour the milk into a pot and warm it to about 21°C.
2. Add the cultured buttermilk and stir well.
3. Pour the mixture into a clean jar.
4. Cover with a lid and let stand at room temperature for 12-24 hours, until the milk has thickened and has a sour taste.
5. Place the buttermilk in the refrigerator and serve cold. It can be stored in the refrigerator for up to 2 weeks.

Note:

Storage: Freshly made buttermilk should be stored in the refrigerator and typically lasts about 1 to 2 weeks.

Usage: Buttermilk that has passed its optimum freshness can still be safely used in baking recipes, where the taste is often less noticeable.

Smell and Taste: Fresh buttermilk has a sour taste. An unpleasant or rotten smell is a sign that the buttermilk is no longer good.

10.DIY RECIPES
SKINCARE FOR SENSITIVE SKIN

SENSITIVE SKIN: A BRIEF OVERVIEW

Sensitive skin is often characterized by redness, irritation and an uncomfortable feeling of tightness. It reacts more quickly to external influences such as wind, sun, cold, or cosmetic products. The causes of sensitive skin can be varied, including genetic factors, environmental stressors, or a compromised skin barrier.

Sensitive skin requires special attention and care. It benefits from gentle, moisturizing and anti-inflammatory ingredients that soothe the skin and strengthen its natural barrier function. It is important to avoid harsh ingredients, fragrances and alcohol, as these can further irritate the skin. Instead, products should be chosen that nourish, hydrate and protect the skin without overwhelming it.

Sensitive skin needs gentle care that strengthens the skin barrier, reduces redness and irritation and provides moisture. Fermented ingredients can help soothe the skin and support its natural flora.

Homemade Cosmetics for sensitive skin

Below are recipes for homemade cosmetic products specifically developed for sensitive skin. They include fermented ingredients mentioned in this book and offer soothing care without irritating the skin.

TONICS FOR SENSITIVE SKIN

Tonics, also known as facial waters, are a crucial part of skincare that is often overlooked. These watery solutions are applied to the skin after cleansing and before the application of serums and moisturizers. Their purpose is to remove residues from cleansing products, balance the skin's pH and deliver soothing ingredients.
Tonics prove to be particularly beneficial for sensitive skin. These skin types tend to react more sensitively to external influences such as wind, sun, cold, or cosmetic products. They often suffer from redness, irritation and an uncomfortable tightness. Tonics specially formulated for sensitive skin are designed to alleviate these skin issues and provide nourishment.

FERMENTED CHAMOMILE TONIC

This homemade fermented tonic for sensitive skin is a gentle and nurturing addition to your skincare routine. The combination of fermented chamomile extract and aloe vera provides your skin with the soothing and moisturizing it needs.

Ingredients:
- 20g fermented chamomile extract
- 15g Aloe Vera gel (fresh or available with a content of 90-99%)
- 40g rose water (available at drugstores or Turkish supermarkets)

Instructions for preparation:
1. Mix the fermented chamomile extract, Aloe Vera gel and rose water in a clean spray bottle.
2. Close the bottle tightly and shake it well to thoroughly mix the ingredients.
3. Your soothing fermented chamomile tonic for sensitive skin is now ready to use. Store it in the refrigerator to maintain freshness.
4. Keep it refrigerated and use it within 1-2 weeks.

Application: After cleansing the face, spray the tonic onto the face and let it sit briefly to soothe the skin and regulate the pH level. Then apply serum and moisturizer.

FERMENTED LAVENDER TONIC

This homemade fermented tonic for sensitive skin is a soothing addition to your skincare routine. The combination of fermented lavender extract and Aloe Vera provides your skin with the necessary calming and hydration.

Ingredients:
- 25g fermented lavender extract
- 15g Aloe Vera gel (fresh or with a content of 90-99%)
- 40g rose water (available in drugstores or Turkish supermarkets)

Instructions for preparation:
1. Mix the fermented lavender extract, Aloe Vera gel and rose water in a clean spray bottle.
2. Close the bottle tightly and shake it well to thoroughly mix the ingredients.
3. Your gentle fermented lavender tonic for sensitive skin is now ready to use.
4. Store it in the refrigerator and use it within 1-2 weeks.

Application: After cleansing your face, lightly spray the tonic on your face. Let it act briefly to soothe the skin and balance the pH level. Then apply your serum and afterward your moisturizer. Avoid direct contact with the eyes. Gently patting the tonic into the skin promotes absorption and optimally prepares the skin for subsequent care steps.

SERUM FOR SENSITIVE SKIN

Serums provide intensive care for sensitive skin by delivering targeted hydration and soothing irritation. Their lightweight formulation allows deep penetration to deliver nourishing ingredients directly to the skin cells without causing irritation. Formulated with ingredients like Aloe Vera and green tea extract, they strengthen the skin barrier and calm sensitive skin. A serum can soothe the skin, provide hydration and promote balanced skin tone.

FERMENTED GREEN TEA SERUM

This homemade fermented tonic for sensitive skin is a gentle and nurturing addition to your skincare routine. The combination of fermented green tea extract and Aloe Vera provides your skin with the necessary calming and moisture.

Ingredients:
- 20g fermented green tea extract
- 10g natural yogurt (homemade or store-bought)
- 15g Aloe Vera gel
- 5g fermented ginseng extract
- Lavender essential oil (2-3 drops)

Instructions for preparation::
1. Mix the fermented green tea extract and Aloe Vera gel in a clean bowl.
2. Add the yogurt and stir well.
3. Add the fermented ginseng extract and mix again.
4. Finally, add 2-3 drops of lavender essential oil and stir until well combined.
5. Transfer the serum to a clean bottle or container. Store it in the refrigerator and use it within 1-2 weeks.

Application: Apply the serum morning and evening after cleansing and using the tonic and before applying moisturizer to your face. Avoid the eye area. Gently pat into the skin until fully absorbed.

FERMENTED JOJOBA OIL SERUM

This carefully formulated serum combines fermented jojoba oil and chamomile extract with koji rice extract to gently nourish sensitive skin. While chamomile has soothing properties, jojoba oil provides deep hydration. Koji rice extract enriches the formula with its antioxidant properties, supports the skin barrier and promotes healthy skin moisture, making it especially valuable for sensitive skin types.

Ingredients:
- 5g fermented jojoba oil
- 20g fermented chamomile extract
- 10g kefir
- 15g fermented koji rice extract
- Essential rose oil (2-3 drops)

Instructions for preparation:
1. Mix the fermented chamomile extract and the fermented koji rice extract in a clean bowl.
2. Add the kefir and stir well.
3. Add the jojoba oil and mix again.
4. Finally, add 2-3 drops of rose oil and stir until well combined.
5. Transfer the serum to a clean bottle or container. Store it in the refrigerator and use it within 1-2 weeks.

Application: Apply the serum morning and evening after cleansing and using the tonic and before applying moisturizer to your face. Avoid the eye area. Gently pat into the skin until fully absorbed.

MOISTURIZER FOR SENSITIVE SKIN

Moisturizers provide essential care for sensitive skin by deeply hydrating and strengthening the skin barrier. Their carefully selected formulations are designed to intensively nourish the skin without causing irritation. It is an essential part of the daily morning and evening skincare routine, especially for those with sensitive skin.

SOOTHING GREEN TEA HARMONY CREAM

This soothing cream combines the nurturing properties of fermented chamomile extract and fermented green tea extract with the moisturizing benefits of fermented jojoba oil and shea butter. The addition of fermented rose extract gives the cream a delicate scent and completes the skincare experience.

Ingredients:
- 5g fermented chamomile extract
- 10g fermented jojoba oil
- 5g fermented green tea extract
- 2g shea butter
- 2-3 drops of fermented rose extract

Instructions for preparation:
1. Melt the shea butter: Use a water bath to gently melt the shea butter.
2. Combine the oils and extracts: Add the fermented jojoba oil, the fermented green tea extract and the fermented chamomile extract to the melted shea butter and stir well.
3. Add the fermented rose extract: Add the drops of rose extract and stir again to obtain a homogeneous cream.
4. Fill and cool: Transfer the cream into a clean container and let it cool completely.

Application: Apply the cream morning and evening after cleansing, using the tonic and any serums. Gently massage a small amount into the skin until fully absorbed. This cream provides intense hydration and leaves the skin feeling soothed and balanced. Store it in the refrigerator and use it within 1-2 weeks to ensure freshness.

GENTLE LAVENDER BALANCE CREAM

This gently nurturing cream utilizes the soothing properties of fermented lavender extract and combines them with the moisturizing effects of fermented bamboo extract. Fermented kombu extract adds antioxidant benefits and supports the skin barrier, making the cream especially valuable for sensitive skin types.

Ingredients:

- 10g fermented lavender extract
- 10g fermented bamboo extract
- 5g Aloe Vera gel (fermented if available)
- 5g fermented kombu extract (seaweed)
- 3g fermented jojoba oil
- 1-2 drops of fermented rose extract

Instructions for preparation::

1. Mix the extracts: Combine the fermented lavender extract, fermented bamboo extract, and fermented kombu extract in a clean bowl.
2. Add Aloe Vera gel and jojoba oil: Stir in the Aloe Vera gel and fermented jojoba oil to enhance the moisturizing properties.
3. Add the fermented rose extract.
4. Homogenize: Stir the mixture well until a uniform cream is achieved.
5. Fill and cool: Transfer the cream into a clean container and let it cool until it sets.

Application: Apply the cream morning and evening after cleansing, using the tonic and any serums. Gently massage a small amount into the skin until fully absorbed. This cream provides deep hydration and leaves the skin feeling soothed and balanced. Store it in the refrigerator and use it within 1-2 weeks to ensure optimal freshness.

11.DIY RECIPES SKINCARE FOR OILY SKIN

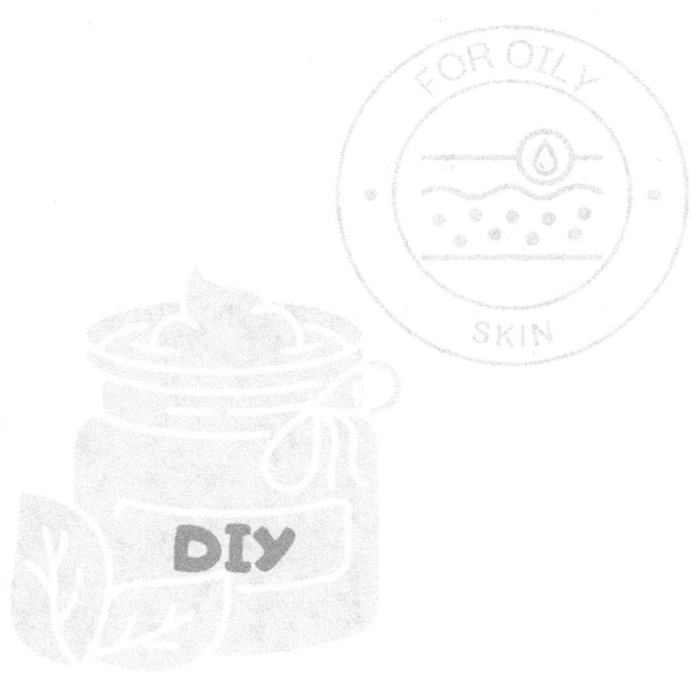

OILY SKIN: A BRIEF OVERVIEW

Oily skin is characterized by increased shine, enlarged pores and a tendency towards blemishes and acne. These skin types produce excess sebum, often influenced by hormonal fluctuations or genetic factors. A common misconception is that oily skin needs drying care, in fact, this can stimulate further sebum production.

It is essential to provide oily skin with adequate moisture to balance the sebum and not stimulate overproduction of oil. Traditional Asian fermentation cosmetics offer ideal solutions for this. Fermented ingredients such as green tea, rice water and ginseng are naturally moisturizing and soothing without clogging pores. These ingredients help calm the skin and support its natural barrier function, making them particularly effective for oily skin types.

Homemade cosmetics for oily skin

Below are recipes specifically designed for oily skin that include fermented ingredients. These recipes utilize the natural properties of Asian ferments to effectively care for the skin and improve the appearance of shine and blemishes without irritating the skin.

TONICS FOR OILY SKIN

Tonics, an essential part of the daily skincare routine, are particularly important for the care of oily skin. These aqueous solutions are used after facial cleansing and before the application of serums and moisturizers. They serve to remove excess oil and residues from cleansing products, normalize the skin's pH level and simultaneously provide skin-soothing ingredients.

Tonics are greatly beneficial for oily skin as they help regulate excess sebum without drying out the skin. Ingredients such as fermented green tea and koji rice, commonly used in Asian fermentation cosmetics, not only cleanse the skin but also soothe it and strengthen its barrier function.

FERMENTED GREEN TEA TONIC

This homemade fermented tonic is ideal for oily skin, as green tea is known for its astringent and pore-refining properties. It helps control excess sebum and clarify the complexion.

Ingredients:
- 30g fermented green tea extract
- 20g witch hazel water (available in drugstores or pharmacies, known for its anti-inflammatory and pore-minimizing effects)

Instructions for preparation::
1. Mix the fermented green tea extract and witch hazel water in a clean spray bottle.
2. Close the bottle tightly and shake well to thoroughly mix the ingredients.
3. Store the tonic in the refrigerator to maintain freshness.
4. Use it morning and evening after cleansing and before applying other skincare products.

Application: After facial cleansing, spray the tonic on the face and let it act for a short while to soothe the skin and regulate the pH level. Then apply serum and moisturizer.

FERMENTED RICE WATER TONIC

Fermented rice water is rich in vitamins and minerals that nourish the skin, while also balancing oil production and brightening the complexion.

Ingredients:
- 40g fermented rice water
- 10g cucumber water
- 2-3 drops of tea tree oil (antibacterial)

Instructions for preparation::
1. Combine the fermented rice water and cucumber water in a clean spray bottle.
2. Add 2-3 drops of tea tree oil. Make sure to dilute the oil well to avoid skin irritation.
3. Shake the bottle vigorously to mix all the ingredients thoroughly.
4. Store the tonic in the refrigerator to maintain optimal freshness.
5. Spray the tonic on the skin after facial cleansing and let it dry naturally before applying further skincare products.

Application: After facial cleansing, lightly spray the tonic on your face. Let it act briefly to soothe the skin and balance the pH level. Then apply your serum and afterward your moisturizer. Avoid direct contact with the eyes. Gently patting the tonic into the skin promotes absorption and optimally prepares the skin for subsequent care steps.

SERUM FOR OILY SKIN

Serums provide intensive care for oily skin by specifically controlling excess sebum and refining pores. Their lightweight formulation allows for deep penetration to deliver nourishing ingredients directly to the skin cells without clogging pores. Formulated with ingredients like fermented kombu and green tea extract, they help clarify the skin and reduce excess shine. A serum can mattify the skin, reduce pore size and ensure a balanced complexion.

KOMBU AND GREEN TEA SERUM

This homemade fermented serum for oily skin is a valuable addition to your skincare routine. The combination of fermented kombu extract and green tea provides your skin with the needed clarification and control over sebum.

Ingredients:
- 20g fermented kombu extract
- 20g fermented green tea extract
- 10g Aloe Vera gel
- 5g fermented black rice extract
- Essential tea tree oil (1-2 drops)

Instructions for preparation::
1. Mix the fermented kombu extract and Aloe Vera gel in a clean bowl.
2. Add the green tea extract and stir well.
3. Add the fermented black rice extract and mix again.
4. Finally, add 1-2 drops of tea tree oil and stir until well mixed.
5. Transfer the serum into a clean bottle or container. Store it in the refrigerator and use it within 1-2 weeks.

Application: Apply the serum morning and evening after cleansing and using the tonic and before applying moisturizer to your face. Avoid the eye area. Gently pat into the skin until fully absorbed.

SOYBEAN AND KEFIR SERUM

This carefully formulated serum combines fermented soybean extract (Cheonggukjang), kefir and fermented black rice extract to nourish and balance oily skin. Soybean extract is known for its antioxidant and moisturizing properties that help nourish the skin while controlling excess sebum. Kefir, rich in probiotics, supports the skin microbiome and promotes healthy skin flora. Black rice extract provides additional antioxidant benefits and helps soothe and protect the skin.

Ingredients:
- 15g fermented soybean extract
- 10g kefir
- 10g fermented black rice extract
- 5g fermented jojoba oil
- Essential lavender oil (2-3 drops)

Instructions for preparation:
1. Mix the fermented soybean extract and fermented black rice extract in a clean bowl.
2. Add kefir and stir well to integrate the probiotic properties.
3. Add the fermented jojoba oil and mix again.
4. Finally, add 2-3 drops of lavender oil and stir until well mixed.
5. Transfer the serum into a clean bottle or container. Store it in the refrigerator and use it within 1-2 weeks.

Application: Apply the serum morning and evening after cleansing and using the tonic and before applying moisturizer to your face. Avoid the eye area. Gently pat into the skin until fully absorbed. This serum helps soothe, hydrate, and balance the skin while promoting a fresh, clear complexion.

MOISTURIZER FOR OILY SKIN

Moisturizers are crucial for caring for oily skin by providing hydration without clogging pores or weighing down the complexion. An effective moisturizer for oily skin uses light, water-based formulations that refresh and nourish the skin.

LIGHT HYDRO-BALANCE CREAM

This lightweight moisturizer is specially formulated for oily skin and combines refreshing aloe vera juice with the balancing properties of fermented koji rice extract and fermented jujube extract.

Ingredients:
- 15g aloe vera juice
- 10g fermented koji rice extract
- 5g fermented jujube extract
- 3g hyaluronic acid powder (sodium hyaluronate - available online)
- 0.5g xanthan gum thickener (available online)
- 70g distilled water or rose water
- 1-2 drops of fermented rose extract

Instructions for preparation:
1. Prepare the water base: In a clean pot or bowl, mix the distilled water or rose water with aloe vera juice. Heat the mixture slightly without boiling to create a uniform base.
2. Dissolve the hyaluronic acid: Add the hyaluronic acid and stir continuously until fully dissolved. This can take a few minutes as hyaluronic acid sometimes hydrates slowly.
3. Add the xanthan gum: Slowly sprinkle the xanthan gum into the mixture while continuously stirring to avoid lumps. Continue stirring until the mixture slightly thickens and takes on a gel-like consistency.
4. Add the fermented koji rice extract, rose extract, and fermented jujube extract. Stir thoroughly to ensure all ingredients are evenly distributed.
5. Homogenize: Stir the mixture smoothly to avoid lumps.
6. Let the mixture cool to room temperature. Then transfer the finished cream into a clean, sterilized container with a tight-fitting lid and store it in the refrigerator.

REVITALIZING KOMBU & BAMBOO CREAM

This refreshing moisturizer combines the antioxidant benefits of fermented kombu extract with the intense hydration of fermented bamboo extract. Additionally, fermented soybean extract helps to nourish and balance the skin, making this cream particularly valuable for oily skin types.

Ingredients:
- 110g fermented kombu extract (seaweed)
- 10g fermented bamboo extract
- 5g fermented soybean extract
- 3g hyaluronic acid (low molecular weight)
- 0.5g xanthan gum
- 70g distilled water or rose water
- 1-2 drops of fermented rose extract

Instructions for preparation::
1. Prepare the water base: Gently heat the distilled water or rose water in a clean pot without boiling.
2. Dissolve hyaluronic acid and xanthan gum: Slowly sprinkle the xanthan gum and hyaluronic acid into the warmed water, continuously stirring to avoid clumping. Stir until the mixture achieves a uniform, gel-like consistency.
3. Incorporate extracts: Add the fermented kombu extract, bamboo extract, and soybean extract. Stir thoroughly to ensure a homogeneous mixture.
4. Add fragrance: Add 1-2 drops of the fermented rose extract and stir well.
5. Cool and bottle: Let the mixture cool before transferring it to a clean, sterilized container.

Application: Apply the cream morning and evening after cleansing and a suitable tonic. Gently massage a small amount into the skin until fully absorbed. This light, water-based cream provides intense hydration without clogging pores or leaving a greasy feel. Ideal for oily skin prone to blemishes. Store the cream in the refrigerator and use it within 1-2 weeks to ensure optimal freshness and efficacy.

12.DIY RECIPES
SKINCARE FOR DRY SKIN

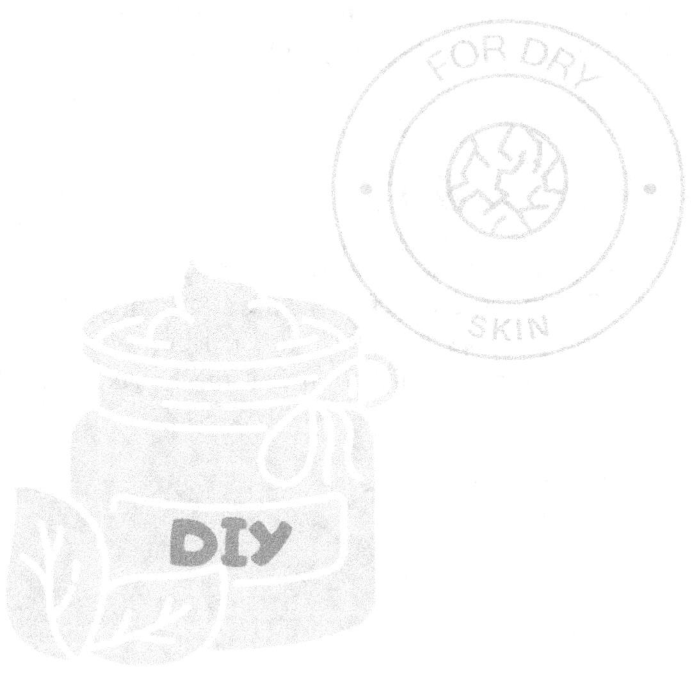

DRY SKIN: A BRIEF OVERVIEW

Dry skin is often characterized by a tight, rough feel and tends to flake, redden and become irritated. This skin type does not produce enough sebum, which weakens the natural protective barrier of the skin, making it more susceptible to environmental influences. Many people try to treat dry skin with rich, often too heavy creams, which do not always address the underlying problems of moisture binding and regulation.

Adequate hydration is crucial to keep the skin supple and strengthen the barrier function. Asian fermentation cosmetics offer excellent solutions for dry skin. Fermented ingredients such as bamboo extract, soybeans and jujube provide deep hydration and support skin renewal. These ingredients are rich in antioxidants and natural emollients that penetrate deeply into the skin and provide lasting moisture without clogging pores.

Homemade cosmetics for dry skin

Below are recipes for homemade cosmetic products specifically developed for dry skin. These utilize the special properties of fermented Asian ingredients to intensely nourish and hydrate the skin. The recipes aim to soothe the skin, provide moisture, and strengthen the natural protective barrier to promote a soft and balanced skin feel.

TONICS FOR DRY SKIN

Tonics, an essential part of the daily skincare routine, are particularly important for the care of dry skin. These aqueous solutions are used after facial cleansing and before the application of serums and moisturizers. They serve to remove residues from cleansing products, balance the skin's pH and simultaneously provide intensely hydrating ingredients.

Tonics are very beneficial for dry skin as they help lock in moisture deep within the skin while also soothing it. Ingredients like fermented bamboo extract and rose extract, commonly used in Asian fermentation cosmetics, not only intensely hydrate the skin but also nourish it and strengthen its barrier function.

FERMENTED GREEN TEA TONIC

This homemade fermented tonic is ideal for dry skin, as rose extract is known for its intense moisturizing and skin-soothing properties. It helps to nourish, calm and hydrate the skin.

Ingredients:
- 30g fermented rose extract
- 20g Aloe Vera gel

Instructions for preparation:
1. Mix the ingredients: Combine the fermented rose extract and the Aloe Vera gel in a clean spray bottle.
2. Shake well: Seal the bottle and shake vigorously to ensure that the ingredients are thoroughly mixed.
3. Keep cool: Store the tonic in the refrigerator to preserve the freshness and effective properties of the ingredients.
4. Application: Use the tonic morning and evening after cleansing. Lightly spray it on the face and gently pat it in to promote absorption before applying further skincare products.

Application: After cleansing, spray the tonic onto your face and let it sit briefly to soothe the skin and regulate the pH level. Afterwards, apply serum and moisturizer.

FERMENTED GREEN TEA TONIC

This homemade tonic is specially designed for dry skin, harnessing the moisturizing properties of yogurt to nourish and hydrate the skin. The lactic acid components of yogurt help soothe the skin and reduce the appearance of dryness.

Ingredients:
- 40g fermented yogurt
- 20g aloe vera gel (fermented, if available)
- 5g fermented black rice extract
- 2-3 drops of lavender oil (for a soothing scent and additional care)

Instructions for preparation:
1. Mix the ingredients: Add the fermented yogurt, aloe vera gel and fermented black rice extract into a clean spray bottle.
2. Add the essential oil: Include 2-3 drops of lavender oil to give the mixture a pleasant scent and provide additional nurturing properties.
3. Shake well: Seal the bottle and shake vigorously to ensure all ingredients are well mixed.
4. Store cool: Keep the tonic refrigerated to preserve its freshness and enhance its refreshing properties.

Application: After facial cleansing, lightly spray the tonic on the face. Let it sit briefly to soothe and moisturize the skin. Then apply your serum and moisturizer to lock in the active ingredients and optimally care for the skin. Avoid direct contact with the eyes and do not spray the tonic into the eyes. Gently patting the tonic onto the skin will enhance absorption and prepare the skin for subsequent care steps.

SERUM FOR DRY SKIN

Serums play a crucial role in the care of dry skin by providing targeted hydration and strengthening the skin barrier. Their lightweight formulation allows for deep penetration to intensely nourish the skin without weighing it down. Formulated with ingredients such as fermented rice water and coconut oil, they help moisturize the skin and make it supple. A serum can soothe the skin, relieve dryness and promote a balanced complexion.

RICE WATER AND COCONUT OIL SERUM

This serum for dry skin is a valuable addition to your skincare routine. The combination of fermented rice water and coconut oil provides the necessary moisture and care for your skin.

Ingredients:
- 20g fermented rice water
- 15g fermented coconut oil
- 10g aloe vera gel
- 5g fermented black rice extract
- Essential lavender oil (1-2 drops)

Instructions for preparation:
1. Mix the fermented rice water and aloe vera gel in a clean bowl.
2. Add the fermented coconut oil and stir well.
3. Add the fermented black rice extract and mix again.
4. Finally, add 1-2 drops of lavender oil and stir until well blended.
5. Transfer the serum to a clean bottle or container. Store it in the refrigerator and use within 1-2 weeks.

Application: Apply the serum in the morning and evening after cleansing and toning and before moisturizing your face. Avoid the eye area. Gently pat the serum into the skin until fully absorbed.

ROSE AND YOGURT SERUM

This carefully curated serum combines the moisturizing properties of rose extract and yogurt to intensely nourish and soothe dry skin. Rose extract is rich in antioxidants and has anti-inflammatory properties that help calm and protect the skin. Yogurt contains lactic acid, which gently exfoliates and moisturizes the skin.

Ingredients:
- 15g fermented rose extract
- 15g yogurt
- 10g fermented pomegranate extract
- 5g fermented kelp extract
- 2-3 drops of lavender essential oil

Instructions for preparation:
1. Mix the fermented rose extract and yogurt in a clean bowl.
2. Add the fermented pomegranate extract and fermented kelp extract.
3. Add 2-3 drops of lavender essential oil and stir well until a uniform mixture is formed.
4. Transfer the serum into a clean bottle or container.
5. Store it in a cool, dry place and use it within 1-2 weeks.

Application: Apply the serum morning and evening after cleansing and toning and before moisturizing the face. Avoid the eye area. Gently pat into the skin until fully absorbed. This serum helps intensely moisturize and soothe the skin, leaving it soft, supple and radiant. Use it regularly for best results.

MOISTURIZER FOR DRY SKIN

Moisturizers play a crucial role in caring for dry skin by intensely hydrating and strengthening the skin barrier to prevent moisture loss. An effective moisturizer for dry skin should be rich yet lightweight to adequately nourish the skin and leave a comfortable feeling.

LIGHT HYDRO-BALANCE CREAM

This lightweight moisturizer is specially formulated for dry skin, providing balanced care that intensely hydrates without weighing down the skin. With a delicate blend of fermented rose and lavender extracts along with fermented jojoba oil, the skin is nourished and soothed, while hyaluronic acid ensures optimal moisture balance.

Ingredients:
- 15g fermented rose extract
- 10g fermented lavender extract
- 5g fermented jojoba oil
- 3g hyaluronic acid powder (sodium hyaluronate - available online)
- 0.5g xanthan gum thickening agent (available online)
- 70g distilled water or rose water

Instructions for preparation:
1. Preparing the water base: Mix the distilled water or rose water with the fermented rose and lavender extracts in a clean pot or bowl. Heat the mixture gently without boiling to create a uniform base.
2. Dissolving the hyaluronic acid: Add the hyaluronic acid powder and stir continuously until fully dissolved. This may take a few minutes as hyaluronic acid hydrates slowly.
3. Adding the xanthan gum: Slowly sprinkle the xanthan gum into the mixture while stirring continuously to avoid clumping. Continue stirring until the mixture slightly thickens and takes on a gel-like consistency.
4. Add the fermented jojoba oil and stir thoroughly to ensure it is evenly incorporated into the mixture. Allow the mixture to cool at room temperature.
5. Then, transfer the finished cream into a clean, sterilized container with a tightly sealed lid and store it in the refrigerator to maintain freshness.

POMEGRANATE & ROSE MOISTURIZER

This luxurious moisturizer combines the hydrating properties of fermented pomegranate extract with the soothing effect of fermented rose extract. The formula is complemented by the addition of fermented argan oil, which nourishes the skin and gives it a smooth appearance.

Ingredients:

- 10g fermented pomegranate extract
- 10g fermented rose extract
- 5g fermented argan oil
- 3g hyaluronic acid powder (sodium hyaluronate - available online)
- 0.5g xanthan gum thickening agent (available online)
- 70g distilled water or rose water
- 1-2 drops of essential rose oil

Instructions for preparation:

1. Preparing the water base: Gently warm the distilled water or rose water in a clean pot without bringing it to a boil.
2. Dissolve hyaluronic acid and xanthan gum: Slowly add the xanthan gum and hyaluronic acid to the warm water while stirring constantly to avoid clumping. Continue stirring until a smooth, gel-like consistency is achieved.
3. Incorporate extracts: Add the fermented pomegranate extract, rose extract and fermented argan oil. Stir thoroughly to ensure a homogeneous mixture.
4. Add fragrance: Add 1-2 drops of essential rose oil and mix well.
5. Cool and fill: Allow the mixture to cool before transferring it to a clean, sterilized container.

Application: Apply the cream morning and evening after cleansing and applying a suitable tonic to the skin. Massage a small amount gently into the skin until fully absorbed. This rich moisturizer deeply hydrates dry skin, leaving it smooth and radiant. Store the cream in the refrigerator and use it within 1-2 weeks to maintain freshness.

13.DIY RECIPES
SKINCARE FOR COMBINATION SKIN

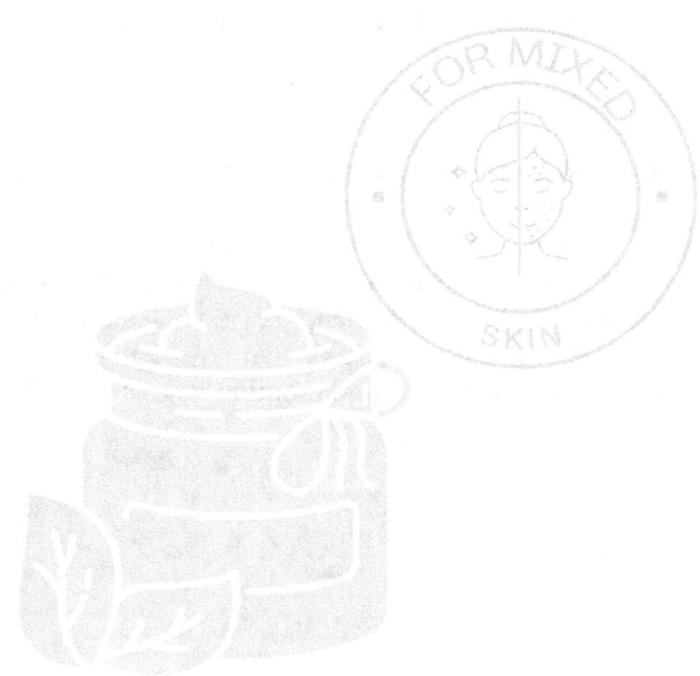

COMBINATION SKIN: A BRIEF OVERVIEW

Combination skin is characterized by a combination of dry and oily areas. While some areas may be dry and rough, others tend to have an oily sheen and may be prone to breakouts. These skin types can be particularly challenging as they have different needs and require specific care to achieve a balance between moisture and oil.

Proper skincare is crucial to balance combination skin and provide it with adequate moisture without overburdening the oily areas. Asian fermentation cosmetics offer excellent solutions for this. Fermented ingredients such as bamboo extract, soybeans and jujube deliver intense hydration while simultaneously supporting the regulation of sebum production. These ingredients are rich in antioxidants and natural emollients that penetrate deeply into the skin, providing long-lasting moisture without clogging the pores.

Homemade cosmetics for combination skin

Below are recipes for homemade cosmetic products specifically tailored to the needs of combination skin. These utilize the unique properties of fermented Asian ingredients to balance the skin, provide moisture and strengthen the natural protective barrier. The recipes aim to soothe the skin, restore the balance between moisture and oil and promote a healthy, radiant complexion.

TONICS FOR COMBINATION SKIN

Tonics play a crucial role in daily skincare routines, especially for combination skin. These watery solutions are used after facial cleansing and before the application of serums and moisturizers. Their goal is to remove residues from cleansing products, balance the skin's pH and provide moisturizing ingredients that meet the needs of combination skin.

Tonics are highly beneficial for combination skin as they help hydrate the skin without overburdening the oily areas. By using ingredients such as fermented green tea extract and lavender extract, which are commonly found in Asian fermentation cosmetics, the skin not only receives intense hydration but also soothing benefits and strengthened natural barrier function.

COMBINATION SKIN BALANCE TONIC

This homemade fermented tonic is an optimal choice for combination skin as it is tailored to the specific needs of this skin type. Bamboo extract provides intense hydration, while chamomile extract soothes and kombu extract nourishes the skin with essential nutrients.

Ingredients:
- 330g fermented bamboo extract
- 20g fermented chamomile extract
- 5g fermented kombu extract (kelp)
- 2 drops of fermented lavender oil (optional)

Instructions for preparation:
1. Mix the fermented bamboo extract, fermented chamomile extract and fermented kombu extract in a clean spray bottle.
2. If desired, add 2 drops of fermented lavender oil to enhance the soothing properties.
3. Seal the bottle tightly and shake it thoroughly to mix all the ingredients well.
4. Store the tonic in the refrigerator to preserve the freshness of the ingredients.

Application: After cleansing the face, lightly spray the tonic onto the face. Allow it to sit briefly before applying your usual moisturizer. Avoid direct contact with the eyes and do not spray the tonic into the eyes.

MOISTURIZING GREEN TEA TONIC

This homemade tonic is perfect for combination skin as it harnesses the refreshing and balancing properties of fermented green tea extract. It helps clarify, soothe and moisturize the skin without overburdening the oily areas.

Ingredients:
- 30g fermented green tea extract
- 20g cucumber water
- 2-3 drops of tea tree oil

Instructions for preparation:
1. Mix the fermented green tea extract and cucumber water in a clean spray bottle.
2. Add 2-3 drops of tea tree oil and thoroughly mix it.
3. Shake the bottle well to combine all the ingredients.
4. Store the tonic in the refrigerator to enhance its refreshing properties.

Application: After cleansing the face, lightly spray the tonic onto the face. Allow it to absorb briefly before applying your usual moisturizer. Avoid direct contact with the eyes and do not spray the tonic into the eyes.

SERUM FOR COMBINATION SKIN

Serums play an important role in skincare for combination skin, as they provide targeted hydration and strengthen the skin barrier. Their light texture allows for effective absorption, nourishing the skin without weighing it down. Serums enriched with fermented ingredients such as green tea extract and jojoba oil aim to hydrate and balance the skin. They help to mattify oily areas while simultaneously nourishing dry spots, supporting a balanced complexion.

GREEN TEA EXTRACT AND JOJOBA OIL SERUM

This serum for combination skin is a targeted addition to your daily routine. The combination of fermented green tea extract and jojoba oil offers the necessary moisture and care for your skin without overwhelming oily areas.

Ingredients:
- 20g fermented green tea extract
- 15g fermented jojoba oil
- 10g aloe vera gel
- 5g fermented kombu extract (seaweed)
- Essential tea tree oil (1-2 drops)

Instructions for preparation:
1. Mix the fermented green tea extract and the aloe vera gel in a clean bowl. Add the fermented jojoba oil and stir thoroughly.
2. Add the fermented kombu extract and mix again.
3. Finally, add 1-2 drops of tea tree oil and stir until everything is well combined. Transfer the serum to a clean bottle or container.
4. Store it in the refrigerator and use within 1-2 weeks.

Application: Apply the serum in the morning and evening after cleansing and toning. Avoid the eye area and gently massage the serum into the skin until fully absorbed.

BALANCING BAMBOO AND SOY SERUM

This serum combines the balancing properties of bamboo extract and soybean extract to intensively care for and balance combination skin. Bamboo extract is known for its hydrating properties and its ability to soothe the skin, while soybean extract helps to nourish and balance the skin.

Ingredients:
- 15g fermented rose extract
- 15g yogurt
- 10g fermented pomegranate extract
- 5g fermented green tea extract
- Essential lavender oil (2-3 drops)

Instructions for preparation:
1. Mix the fermented rose extract and yogurt in a clean bowl.
2. Add the fermented pomegranate extract and fermented green tea extract.
3. Add 2-3 drops of essential lavender oil and stir everything well until the mixture is uniform.
4. Transfer the serum into a clean bottle or container.
5. Store it in a cool, dry place and use within 1-2 weeks.

Application: Apply the serum in the morning and evening after cleansing and toning and before moisturizing. Avoid the eye area. Gently pat the serum into the skin until it is fully absorbed. This serum helps to intensively hydrate and balance the skin. It leaves your skin soft, supple and radiant. Use it regularly for best results.

MOISTURIZER FOR COMBINATION SKIN

Moisturizers are essential for the care of combination skin as they help to hydrate the skin and strengthen its protective layer, promoting a harmonious complexion. An effective moisturizer for combination skin should be lightweight and hydrating without overloading oily areas or promoting impurities.

SOYBEAN BALANCE MOISTURIZER

Enriched with fermented soybean extract, this recipe provides targeted care that hydrates dry skin and mattifies oily areas. Learn how fermented soybeans can hydrate your skin and promote a healthy, balanced appearance.

Ingredients:
- 115g fermented green tea extract
- 10g fermented soybean extract
- 5g fermented jojoba oil
- 3g hyaluronic acid powder (sodium hyaluronate - available online)
- 0.5g xanthan gum thickener (available online)
- 70g distilled water or rose water

Instructions for preparation:
1. Prepare water base: Mix the distilled water or rose water with fermented green tea and soybean extract in a clean pot or bowl. Heat the mixture slightly without boiling to create a uniform base.
2. Dissolve hyaluronic acid: Add the hyaluronic acid powder and stir continuously until it has completely dissolved. This may take a few minutes as the hyaluronic acid hydrates slowly.
3. Add xanthan gum: Gradually sprinkle the xanthan gum into the mixture while continuously stirring to avoid lumps. Continue stirring until the mixture thickens slightly and achieves a gel-like consistency.
4. Integrate fermented jojoba oil: Add the fermented jojoba oil and stir thoroughly to ensure it is evenly incorporated.
5. Cool and bottle: Allow the mixture to cool at room temperature. Then transfer the finished cream into a clean, sterilized container with a tight-fitting lid and store it in the refrigerator to preserve freshness.

GREEN TEA AND CUCUMBER MOISTURIZER

This moisturizer is specially formulated for combination skin, combining the hydrating properties of green tea and chamomile with the soothing effect of cucumber water. It helps to balance and hydrate the skin without overloading oily areas or promoting blemishes. Use it morning and evening after cleansing and toning for optimal care of your combination skin.

Ingredients:

- 15g fermented green tea extract
- 10g fermented chamomile extract
- 5g fermented flaxseed oil
- 3g hyaluronic acid powder (sodium hyaluronate - available online)
- 0.5g xanthan gum thickener (available online)
- 70g distilled water or rose water

Instructions for preparation:

1. Prepare the water base: Mix the distilled water or rose water with the fermented green tea and chamomile extract in a clean pot or bowl. Heat the mixture slightly without boiling to create a uniform base.
2. Dissolve the hyaluronic acid: Add the sodium hyaluronate powder and stir continuously until it has completely dissolved. This may take a few minutes as the hyaluronic acid hydrates slowly.
3. Add the thickener: Gradually sprinkle the xanthan gum into the mixture while continuously stirring to avoid clumping. Continue stirring until the mixture thickens slightly and achieves a gel-like consistency.
4. Integrate the fermented flaxseed oil: Add the fermented flaxseed oil and stir thoroughly to ensure it is evenly incorporated.
5. Cool and bottle: Let the mixture cool at room temperature. Then transfer the finished cream into a clean, sterilized container with a tight-fitting lid and store it in the refrigerator to preserve freshness.

Application: Apply the cream in the morning and evening after cleansing and a suitable tonic. Gently massage a small amount into the skin until fully absorbed. Store the cream in the refrigerator and use it within 1-2 weeks to maintain freshness.

14.DIY RECIPES SKINCARE FOR NORMAL SKIN

NORMAL SKIN: A BRIEF OVERVIEW

Normal skin generally exhibits a balanced ratio of moisture and oil. Although it may seem less demanding, normal skin also requires regular care to maintain its healthy appearance, especially during times of increased stress. Adequate skincare is crucial to optimally support normal skin and keep it well-hydrated, even if it is not as demanding as other skin types. Asian fermentation cosmetics offer excellent solutions for this. Fermented ingredients such as bamboo extract, soybeans and jujube provide intense hydration and help maintain the natural balance of the skin. These ingredients are rich in antioxidants and natural emollients that penetrate deeply into the skin and provide long-lasting moisture without clogging pores.

Homemade Cosmetics for Normal Skin

Below are recipes for homemade cosmetic products specifically tailored to the needs of normal skin. These utilize the unique properties of fermented Asian ingredients to support the skin, provide hydration and strengthen the natural protective barrier. The recipes aim to promote a healthy, radiant complexion and optimally care for the skin during times of increased stress.

TONICS FOR NORMAL SKIN

In the daily skincare routine, tonics play a crucial role, even for normal skin. These aqueous solutions are used after facial cleansing and before the application of serums and moisturizers. Their goal is to remove residues of cleansing products, balance the skin's pH and simultaneously deliver moisturizing ingredients to optimally care for the skin. Tonics are also very beneficial for normal skin as they help hydrate and nourish the skin with essential nutrients.

BALANCING TONIC

This homemade tonic is perfect for normal skin types and provides balancing care. With ingredients like fermented rose extract, aloe vera and green tea, it soothes the skin, hydrates and promotes its natural radiance.

Ingredients:
- 30g fermented rose extract
- 20g aloe vera gel
- 10g fermented green tea extract
- 5g fermented chamomile extract

Instructions for preparation:
1. Mix the fermented rose extract, aloe vera gel, fermented green tea extract and fermented chamomile extract in a clean spray bottle.
2. Seal the bottle and shake vigorously to ensure all ingredients are well mixed.
3. Store the tonic in the refrigerator to preserve the freshness of the ingredients.

Application: After facial cleansing, lightly spray the tonic on the face. Allow it to settle briefly to soothe and hydrate the skin. Then apply your usual care products to lock in the active ingredients and optimally care for the skin. Avoid direct contact with the eyes and do not spray the tonic into the eyes.

FRESH BOOST TONIC

This refreshing tonic for normal skin types is a wonderful addition to your daily skincare routine. With its invigorating blend of fermented green tea extract, cucumber water and mint oil, it hydrates and revitalizes the skin to promote a healthy glow.

Ingredients:
- 30g fermented green tea extract
- 20g cucumber water
- 10g rose water
- 2-3 drops of essential mint oil

Instructions for preparation:
1. Mix the fermented green tea extract, cucumber water and rose water in a clean spray bottle.
2. Add 2-3 drops of essential mint oil to achieve a refreshing scent and provide additional invigorating properties.
3. Seal the bottle tightly and shake well to thoroughly mix all the ingredients.
4. Store the tonic in the refrigerator to preserve freshness and enhance its refreshing properties.

Application: Spray the tonic on the skin after facial cleansing and let it dry naturally. Use it in the morning and evening or as needed to refresh and moisturize your skin. Be sure to shake it well before use. Avoid direct contact with the eyes and do not spray the tonic into the eyes.

SERUM FOR NORMAL SKIN

Proper care is just as important for normal skin as it is for any other skin type. Serums are indispensable aids in optimally hydrating the skin and keeping it healthy and radiant. With their light texture, they provide intensive care without burdening the skin. This special serum, enriched with moisturizing ingredients such as hyaluronic acid and vitamins, is perfectly suited to pamper normal skin and give it a fresh, youthful appearance.

SOOTHING LAVENDER SERUM

This soothing serum for normal skin is an ideal addition to your daily skincare routine. Enriched with fermented lavender extract and fermented black rice extract, it offers intense moisture and gently nourishes the skin.

Ingredients:
- 20g fermented lavender extract
- 15g fermented black rice extract
- 10g fermented jojoba oil
- 5g fermented soybean extract
- Essential rose oil (1-2 drops)
-

Instructions for preparation:
1. Mix the fermented lavender extract and fermented black rice extract in a clean bowl.
2. Add the fermented jojoba oil and stir thoroughly.
3. Add the fermented soybean extract and mix again.
4. Finally, add 1-2 drops of essential rose oil and stir until well blended.
5. Transfer the serum to a clean bottle or container. Store it in a cool place and use it within 1-2 weeks.

Application: Apply the serum in the morning and evening after cleansing to the face. Gently massage it into the skin until fully absorbed. Avoid contact with the eye area.

MOISTURIZING ROSE SERUM

This hydrating rose serum is perfect for normal skin. It combines fermented rose extract with fermented green tea extract to provide intense moisture and revitalize the skin.

Ingredients:

- 20g fermented rose extract
- 15g fermented green tea extract
- 10g aloe vera gel
- 5g fermented jojoba oil
- Essential lavender oil (1-2 drops)

Instructions for preparation:

1. Mix the fermented rose extract and fermented green tea extract in a clean bowl.
2. Add the aloe vera gel and stir well.
3. Add the fermented jojoba oil and mix thoroughly.
4. Finally, add 1-2 drops of essential lavender oil and stir until well blended.
5. Transfer the serum to a dark bottle or container. Store it in a cool, dark place and use it within 4-6 weeks.

Application: Apply the rose serum in the morning and evening after cleansing and toning the face. Gently massage a small amount into the skin until fully absorbed. This serum provides intense hydration and leaves the skin soft and supple.

MOISTURIZER FOR NORMAL SKIN

Moisturizers play a crucial role in daily skincare, even for normal skin, to provide adequate hydration and strengthen the skin barrier. Our 'Soybean Balance Moisturizer for Normal Skin' offers a light yet rich formula that optimally cares for your skin and leaves a comfortable feel. Although normal skin is less sensitive than other skin types, it still requires proper care to keep it healthy and radiant.

REVITALIZING GINSENG CREAM

The revitalizing Ginseng Green Tea Moisturizer combines the power of fermented ginseng and green tea extract with the luxurious feel of argan oil. This rich yet lightweight formula helps hydrate the skin and give it a radiant, youthful appearance.

Ingredients:

- 15g fermented ginseng extract
- 10g fermented green tea extract
- 5g fermented argan oil
- 3g hyaluronic acid powder (sodium hyaluronate - available online)
- 0.5g xanthan gum thickener (available online)
- 70g distilled water or rose water

Instructions for preparation:

1. Mix the distilled water or rose water with the fermented ginseng and green tea extract in a pot or bowl. Heat the mixture slightly without boiling to create a uniform base.
2. Dissolve the hyaluronic acid: Add the hyaluronic acid powder and stir continuously until it has completely dissolved. This may take a few minutes as the hyaluronic acid hydrates slowly.
3. Gradually sprinkle the xanthan gum into the mixture while continuously stirring to avoid clumping. Continue stirring until the mixture thickens slightly and achieves a gel-like consistency.
4. Add the fermented argan oil and stir thoroughly to ensure it is evenly incorporated.
5. Let the mixture cool at room temperature. Then transfer the finished cream into a clean, sterilized container with a tight-fitting lid and store it in the refrigerator to preserve freshness.

SOOTHING CUCUMBER MOISTURIZER

This soothing and nourishing moisturizer is specially formulated for normal skin. It combines the refreshing properties of cucumber water with the moisturizing effects of aloe vera and the revitalizing impact of fermented rose extract. Use this cream daily to hydrate your skin and promote a radiant, healthy appearance.

Ingredients:

- 15g fermented rose extract
- 10g aloe vera gel
- 5g cucumber water
- 3g hyaluronic acid powder (sodium hyaluronate - available online)
- 0.5g xanthan gum thickener (available online)
- 70g distilled water or cucumber water

Instructions for preparation:

1. Mix the distilled water or cucumber water with the fermented rose extract in a clean pot or bowl. Heat the mixture slightly without boiling to create a uniform base.
2. Add the hyaluronic acid powder and stir continuously until it has completely dissolved.
3. Gradually sprinkle the xanthan gum into the mixture while continuously stirring to avoid clumping. Continue stirring until the mixture thickens slightly and achieves a gel-like consistency.
4. Integrate the fermented cucumber water and aloe vera gel into the mixture and stir thoroughly until all ingredients are well mixed.
5. Let the cream cool at room temperature and then transfer it into a clean, sterilized container with a tight-fitting lid. Store the cream in the refrigerator to preserve its freshness and use it daily for smooth, hydrated skin.

Application: Apply the cream in the morning and evening after cleansing and a suitable tonic. Gently massage a small amount into the skin until fully absorbed. Store the cream in the refrigerator and use it within 1-2 weeks to maintain freshness.

15.PATCH TEST

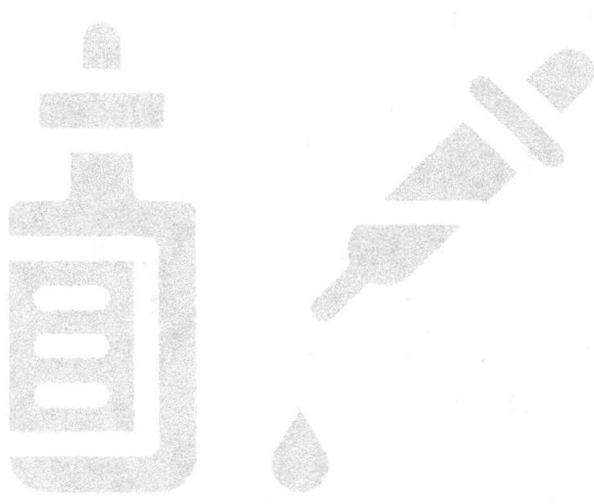

INSTRUCTIONS FOR PATCH TEST

Before using a new cosmetic product containing fermented ingredients, we recommend performing a patch test to ensure that your skin reacts well to it. Follow these steps to conduct the test correctly:

- Clean the Skin: Choose a small spot on the inside of your forearm or behind your ear. Wash the area with water and mild soap, then dry it off.

- Apply the Product: Apply a small amount of the product to the cleaned skin area. It should be enough to lightly cover the area without rubbing it in.

- Wait: Leave the product untouched for 24 hours. Avoid water and intense rubbing in this area during this time.

- Observation: Check the area after 24 hours for signs of a reaction. Look for redness, swelling, itching, or burning.

- Assessment of Results: If no reaction occurs, the product should be safe to use on larger areas. If signs of a reaction appear, thoroughly wash the area with water and mild soap and discontinue use of the product. Consult a dermatologist if necessary.

- Documentation: Record all observations and reactions accurately to refer back to in future product development.

This patch test is an essential step in ensuring the compatibility and safety of cosmetic products, especially those with new or unusual ingredients.

Dear Readers,

Thank you for taking the time to explore "Fermented natural cosmetics - The Power of Microorganisms." Your interest in the traditional techniques and innovations in Asian cosmetics inspires and motivates everyone involved in this project. I hope the book has not only imparted new knowledge but also inspired you to create your own cosmetic formulations. Your support is a valuable encouragement to continue our passion for natural beauty care. Thank you for your purchase and your trust in this work.

With deepest gratitude,

Ava Fiori